NATURAL REMEDIES

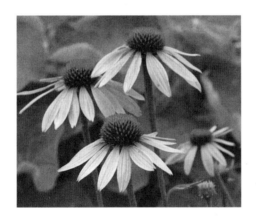

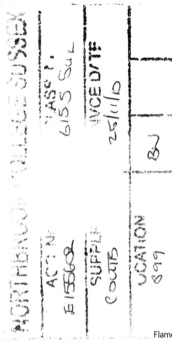

This is a **FLAME TREE** book
First published in 2010

Publisher and Creative Director: Nick Wells
Senior Project Editor: Catherine Taylor
Editorial and Picture Research: Sonya Newland
Art Director: Mike Spender
Layout Design: Dave Jones
Digital Design and Production: Chris Herbert
Proofreader: Tony Phillips
Indexer: Helen Snaith

11 13 14 12 10
1 3 5 7 9 10 8 6 4 2

This edition first published 2010 by
FLAME TREE PUBLISHING
Crabtree Hall, Crabtree Lane
Fulham, London SW6 6TY
United Kingdom

www.flametreepublishing.com

Flame Tree Publishing is part of The Foundry Creative Media Co. Ltd

ISBN 978-1-84786-704-9

A CIP record for this book is available from the British Library upon request.

The author has made all reasonable efforts to ensure that the information in this book is correct at the time of
going to print, and the publishers cannot accept any liability for incorrect or out-of-date information.
The publisher would be glad to rectify any omissions in future editions of this book.

Printed in China

All pictures are courtesy of Shutterstock and © the following photographers:
1 & 54 kanusommer; 3 & 16, 217 matka_Wariatka; 4b & 42 Shanta Giddens; 4t & 46 mtsyri; 5b & 79 Stefano Maccari; 5t & 66, 94 Olga Lipatova;
6b & 110 totalpics; 6b & 95 Viktorus; 6t & 101 Michael C. Gray; 6t & 123 Miodrag Gajic; 8b & 162, 181, 193 Alfred Wekelo; 8t & 202 Vatikaki;
9b & 245 jonphoto; 9t & 238 Palto; 10 & 153, 187 Yuri Arcurs; 11 & 124, 85, 89, 114, 209 Mona Makela; 12 & 199 Jiri Vaclavek; 13 & 156 Kevin Carden;
14 & 30 Irlucik; 15 & 212, 99 Andresr; 18 Vasaleks; 20 ukrphoto; 22 Oleksii Zelivianskyi; 25 marilyn barbone; 27 JuliaSha; 29 Krzysztof Slusarczyk;
32, 247 Sergey Chushkin; 33 Kathie Nichols; 34 Bobby Deal/RealDealPhoto; 37 H. Brauer; 39 Daniel Goodings; 41, 62 LianeM; 45 Dolnikov Denys;
48 Studio Barcelona; 50 readyimage; 51 Santje; 52 Makarova Tatiana; 55 Sergey Ladanov; 58 Gala_Kan; 59 Dale Wagler ; 61 Gyorgy Eger; 64 Iarus;
65 Oleksandr; 67 Robyn Mackenzie; 70 cameilia ; 71 Fanfo; 75 Carsten Medom Madsen; 76 crystalfoto ; 77 Patrycja Müller; 82 Stephanie Frey; 83 Charles B.
Ming Onn; 86 Taratorki; 89 Monika Wisniewska; 90 Damir Karan; 92 michaeljung; 96 Kemeo; 102 Natalia D.; 103, 240 Dusan Zidar; 104 Filipe B. Varela;
105 Danny Smythe; 107 deepblue-photographer; 108 Jozsef Szasz-Fabian; 112 Sven Hoppe; 117 wheatley; 119 michael ledray; 121 Diane N. Ennis;
126 irin-k; 127 Christophe Rolland; 129 Daniel Prudek; 131 Marie C. Fields; 133 Marin; 135 maureen plainfield; 136 Fiona Ayerst; 137 Marek R. Swadzba;
138 dmitriyd; 141 Susan Fox; 142 Steffen Foerster Photography; 145 luSh; 146 Ventin; 149 Lisa F. Young; 150 Christopher Edwin Nuzzaco; 154 Peter Elvidge;
155 Dmitri Mihhailov; 157 Alexander Raths; 159, 185 Monkey Business Images; 160 Holger Mette; 164 Marcel Mooij; 167 MoniV; 168 Marcin Balcerzak;
170 aceshot1; 172 Jeff Davies; 175 Rob Marmion; 176 paul prescott ; 178 Cora Reed; 179 Falko Matte; 183 Nik Frey; 188 Juriah Mosin; 191 Hywit Dimyadi;
195 Worldpics; 197 Christian Wheatley; 200 Konstantin Karchevskiy; 204 Maxim Tupikov; 206 Losevsky Pavel; 210 eAlisa; 214 rongxuan; 218 oknoart;
221 Nic Neish; 222 Larisa Lofitskaya; 225 Nayashkova Olga; 227 sbarabu; 229 Pavel Semenov; 231 Liveshot; 232 Vasiliy Koval;
234 Denis Tabler; 237 karbunar; 243 ffolas; 246 lantapix; 248 Melinda Fawver; 250b Mau Horng; 250t Peter Doomen

NATURAL REMEDIES

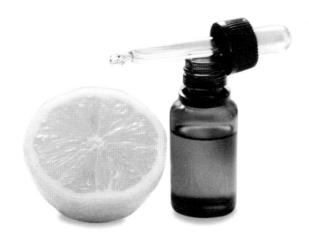

KAREN SULLIVAN
General Editor: TRICIA ALLEN

FLAME TREE
PUBLISHING

Contents

Aromatherapy involves the use of essential oils – the life force of aromatic flowers, herbs, plants, trees or spices, for therapeutic purposes. Each oil has its own natural fragrance and therapeutic action. This chapter covers the main essential oils used in aromatherapy, and explains how they can be applied to the body to improve physical, mental and emotional health.

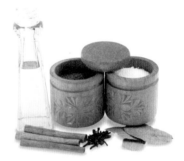

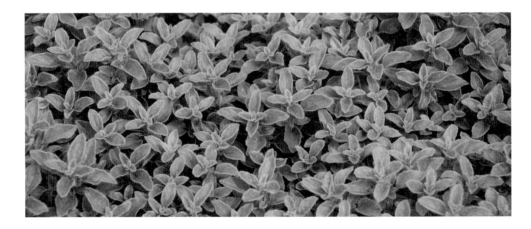

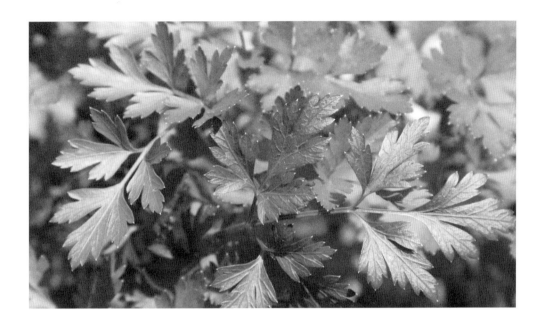

Herbalism

Herbal medicine is designed to be gentle, stimulating our bodies to return to health by strengthening their systems as well as attacking the cause of the illness itself. Extracts are taken from the whole plant (or the whole of a part of the plant, such as the

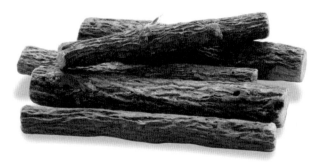

leaves or the roots), not isolated or synthesized to perform specific functions. This chapter explains how the different herbs can be applied to aid holistic healing.

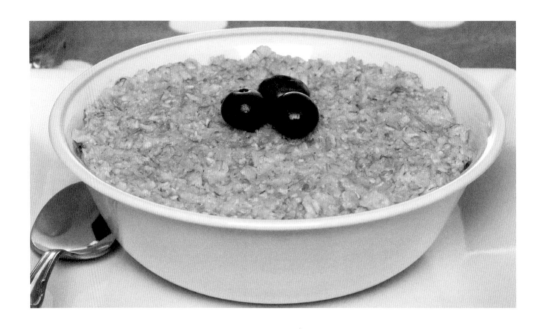

Home Remedies

Until the early part of the twentieth century, every household had a stock of items that could be used to treat minor ailments, including herbs, plants, fruits and various foodstuffs. The use of home remedies is now experiencing a resurgence as people recognize the healing properties of many natural household items. This section explains how to use what's in the larder to treat ailments from cuts and scrapes to colds.

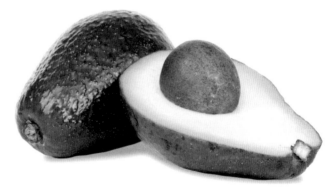

Homeopathy 108

Homeopathy is a system of medicine that supports the body's own healing mechanism, using specially prepared remedies. It is 'energy' medicine, in that it works with the body's vital force to encourage healing and to ensure that all body systems are working at optimum level.

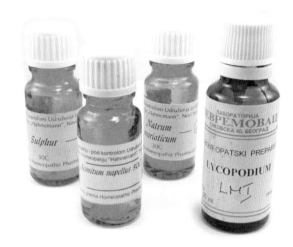

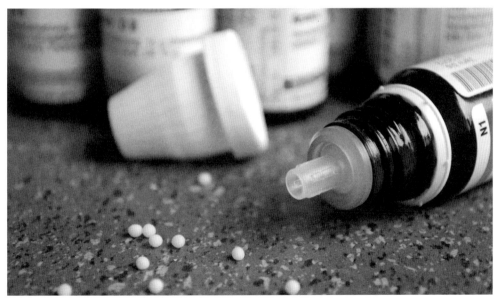

Natural Health 150

Naturopathy is an umbrella term used in most Western countries to cover a range of therapies that come under the heading of natural medicine. This chapter explains how these different therapies – from massage to counselling – work to improve both physical and mental health.

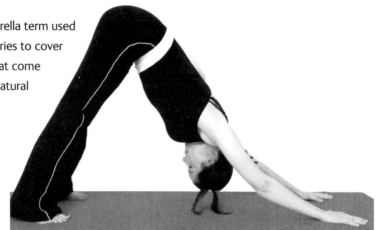

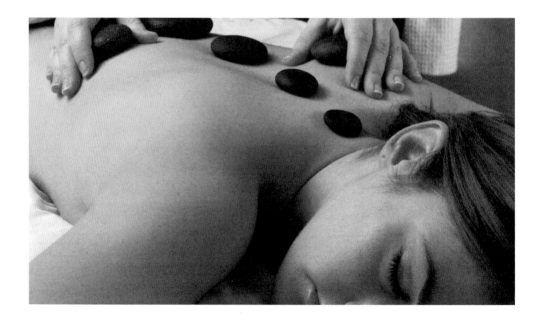

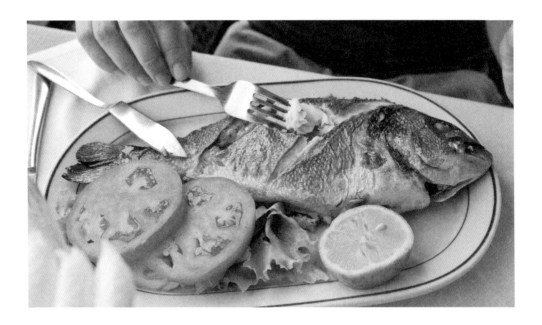

Nutrition 206

A balanced diet is an essential part of a healthy lifestyle, and natural health practitioners have long recommended care in what we eat to both prevent and assist in the recovery of illness. This chapter looks at the importance of having the right vitamins, minerals and other natural products in our diet.

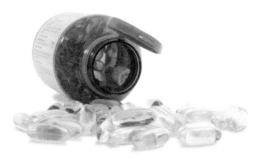

Further Reading & Websites 252
Index 254

Foreword

As the twenty-first century progresses, complementary and alternative medicines are becoming the first preference of health care for many and their popularity is rapidly increasing. Each year, more and more people are choosing to consult a natural-therapy practitioner and the sales of natural remedies are higher than ever before.

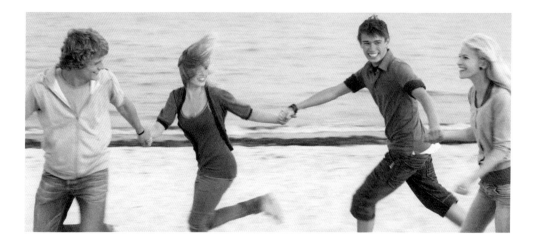

It is not so long ago that natural remedies were the mainstay of medicinal treatment, and this is still the case in many parts of the world. Modern medicine has worked many miracles over the last few decades and few would deny the life-saving properties of modern surgical methods and drugs. Is it possible, however, that in applauding these developments, we have thrown the baby out with the bathwater? Conventional medical approaches have embraced new technologies and the vast array of chemical drugs produced by the pharmaceutical industry, yet have ignored the lessons of the past, which demonstrate that natural therapies and remedies are highly effective in curing many common ailments.

Nowadays many people choose to consult complementary therapists because they are concerned about taking chemical medications and also because they are looking for long-term solutions to their health problems, rather than just short-term relief from the symptoms. I have been a homeopathic practitioner for many years. In that time, I have seen the number of homeopaths in my area increase tenfold, and yet we all achieve busy practices, with approximately 15 to 20 patients every week. The patients who consult me are varied, including pregnant women, parents with young children, businessmen and women, teenagers and the elderly, all with the same desire to be treated holistically with natural remedies.

This book encompasses a wide range of natural remedies: from herbalism to aromatherapy, homeopathy to natural health, nutrition to home remedies. Simple to use, with clear guidelines about the complementary and alternative therapies available today, this book is highly informative and I would have no hesitation in recommending it to anyone with an interest in natural remedies.

Tricia Allen BSc (Hons)
LCH MARH
HOMEOPATH

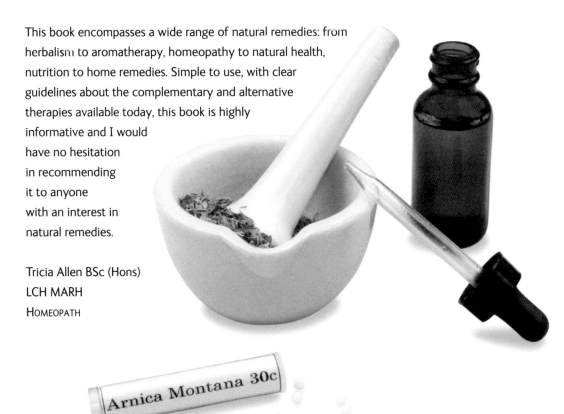

Introduction

Since the beginning of civilization, we have looked to nature to provide us with remedies for healing the body, mind and soul. Throughout time various tribes, communities and societies have had their own healers, methods and medicines, and by using the natural remedies available to them, discovered many effective ways of healing.

Modern Medicine

Until the early part of the twentieth century, every family had a supply of their favourite home remedies, including plants, herbs and foodstuffs that could be used to treat minor medical emergencies, or prevent a common ailment from becoming more serious. The knowledge of how to use these natural remedies was passed down from generation to generation, becoming part of the folklore of each family and community. When illness struck, the cause was investigated and, more often than not, the treatment could be found in the garden, in a field, or in the cupboard.

In the mid-twentieth century, society began to change its outlook towards natural remedies. The advent of modern medicine, with its many miracles, also led to a growing dependency on doctors and an increasingly stretched health-care system. The growth of the pharmaceutical industry has meant that there are indeed palliatives and cures for most disease symptoms, but we have also become accustomed to putting our health completely in the hands of doctors, or instead purchasing medicinal drugs to instantly make

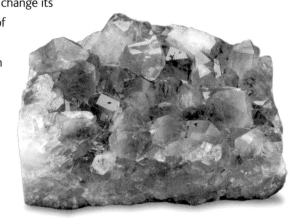

us feel better. We are no longer in touch with our bodies, so when we become ill, we rely on others to treat us. Increasingly, however, we are learning that the conventional medical system is not infallible. Modern medicine may make us feel better in the short term, but it does so by palliating or suppressing the symptoms, not by curing their cause.

Natural Renaissance

The growth in complementary and alternative medicine has been unprecedented. Nearly 20 per cent of the British population regularly use alternative or complementary therapies, including acupuncture, aromatherapy, herbalism, homeopathy and reflexology; spending more than £500 million annually in the process.

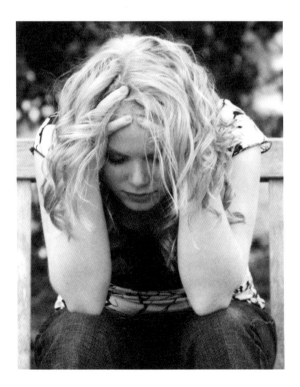

Why the sudden surge of interest in natural remedies? The fact is, that despite conventional medical disdain, there is now a growing body of evidence proving that natural remedies work. In clinical trials comparing drug and herb treatments, some herbs have been coming out on top. For example, it has been proved that St John's wort is as effective as the pharmaceutical antidepressants available to treat mild depression, and there is evidence that large doses of the mineral selenium can protect against cancer.

Our approach to our bodies and to health care in general has changed. People have become tired of the all-too-familiar five-minute consultation with the doctor and also with the prescription that inevitably follows: there are clearly other aspects of patients' lives that need to be taken into consideration. Far from asking questions about emotional health, sleep patterns, diet and exercise, many conventional doctors tend to trot out the old adage 'eat less fat', and bang the symptoms on the head with a drug. Nowadays we expect more. We want to sit down with someone who will listen to us and consider the whole picture, making links between our lifestyle, our past and familial history, the totality of our symptoms and our overall health on every level. This is how the practitioners of complementary and alternative medicine work.

Evaluating the Evidence

The evidence in favour of this approach is overwhelming. Just 30 years ago, the British Medical Journal (BMJ) suggested that complementary medicine 'ought to be as extinct as divination by examination of bird's entrails'. Recently, the BMJ has produced a 12 part series on complementary and alternative medicines. In Europe, complementary medicine plays an important role in preventative and overall health care. In France, one-third of the population use homeopathic medicines and 39 per cent of French family physicians prescribe them. Twenty per cent of all German physicians prescribe homeopathic medicines and 45 per cent of Dutch physicians consider homeopathy an effective form of medicine.

Studies show that many natural therapies and remedies are effective. We are now aware of the positive health benefits of taking supplements, such as antioxidants, and massaging with aromatherapy oils. One study showed that people using acupuncture take 79 per cent fewer prescription drugs, while another showed that asthmatic children were found to improve dramatically within the first few days of taking Ginkgo biloba extract. This is not just a new trend in New Age thinking: natural therapies and remedies offer a safer alternative to conventional medicine, and their efficacy is on the brink of receiving wide scientific support.

A Holistic Approach

Natural therapies are holistic, taking into consideration the mind, body and spirit as equally important elements to good health. Natural remedies work by bringing these three elements into balance, producing a sense of well-being, which in turn allows healing to take place. Even better, natural remedies work to prevent illness, yet treat the cause of disease when it does set in, reducing the duration and possibility of recurrence. As our bodies are literally encouraged to heal themselves, we become stronger, healthier, and more resistant to the rigours of modern-day life.

Natural remedies work on insidious health problems – that are often the result of stress – and have the potential to wipe out a host of niggling health conditions (otherwise an array of medicinal drugs would be needed to help). Why is this the case? Simply because, once the cause is eliminated, symptoms disappear. For example, you can continue to use inhalers for your asthma for years and years, but once you cease the medication, the symptoms return unabated. If you address the cause of your asthma, then you will actually have a good chance of eliminating it once and for all.

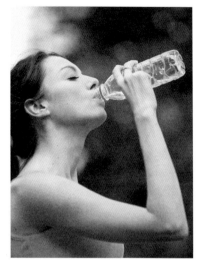

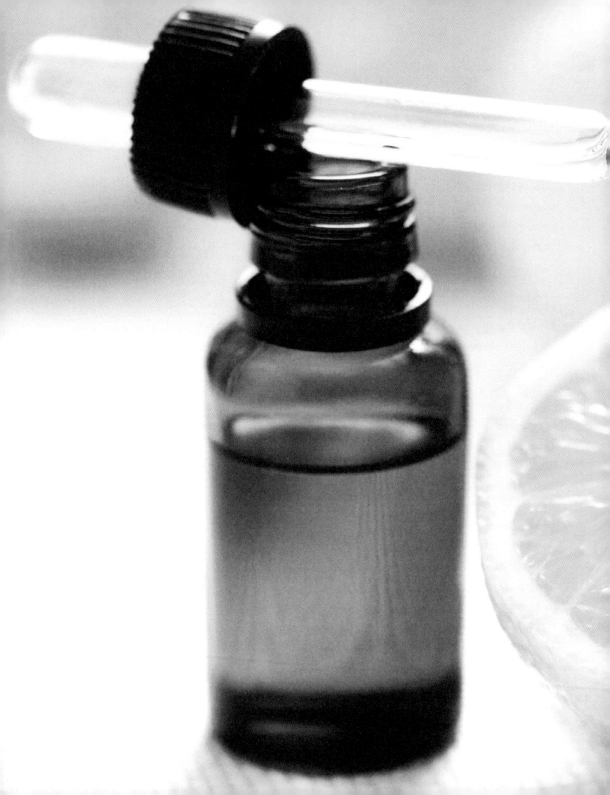

aromatherapy

Understanding Aromatherapy

The word 'aromatherapy' literally means 'treatment using scents', and the therapy has evolved as a branch of herbal medicine. Unlike the herbs used in herbal medicine, essential oils are not taken internally but are inhaled or applied to the skin.

Aromatherapy Treatment

Aromatherapy is gentle enough to be used by people of all ages and states of health. It is nurturing for babies and children and offers comfort and care to the elderly. Pregnant women, and even seriously ill patients can benefit from professional treatment. The therapy has been shown to be particularly effective in preventing and treating stress and anxiety-related disorders, muscular and rheumatic pains, digestive problems, menstrual irregularities, menopausal complaints, insomnia and depression.

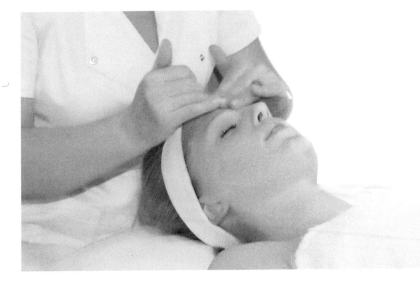

Be Aware

Aromatherapy is compatible with conventional medicine and most other forms of holistic treatment. However, if you are taking other medication, consult your doctor first. Some oils are not compatible with homeopathic treatment. Aromatherapy is safe to use at home for minor or short-term problems providing you follow certain guidelines:

Do not: take essential oils internally unless advised by a registered aromatherapist.

Do not: apply them undiluted to the skin unless it is stated that it is safe to do so.

Do not: put essential oils in the eyes.

Do not: keep essential oils where children can reach them.

Consult a qualified practitioner for advice and treatment if you:

- **Are pregnant**
- **Have an allergy**
- **Have a chronic condition such as high blood pressure or epilepsy**
- **Are receiving medical or psychiatric treatment**
- **Are taking homeopathic remedies**
- **Are treating an infant**

Essential Oils

Essential oils are extracted from the aromatic essences of certain plants, trees, fruit, flowers, herbs and spices. They are natural, volatile oils with identifiable chemical and medicinal properties. Over 150 essential oils have been extracted, each one with its own scent and unique healing properties. Oils are sourced from plants as commonplace as parsley and as exquisite as jasmine. For optimum benefits, essential oils must be extracted from natural raw ingredients and remain as pure as possible.

Essential oils can be used alone or blended together. Oils are blended to create a more sophisticated fragrance or to enhance or change the medicinal actions of the oils. When blended well, therapists can create a synergistic blend, where the oils work in harmony and to great effect.

How Essential Oils Work

Essential oils enter the body by inhalation and absorption through the pores of the skin. Once in the body, they work in three ways: pharmacologically, physiologically and psychologically. The chemical constituents of the oils are carried in the bloodstream to all areas of the body, where they react with the body's chemistry in a way that is similar to drugs. Certain oils also have an affinity with particular areas of the body, and their properties have balancing, sedating or stimulating effects on body systems. Once inhaled, aromatic signals are sent to the limbic system of the brain, where they exert a direct effect on the mind and emotions.

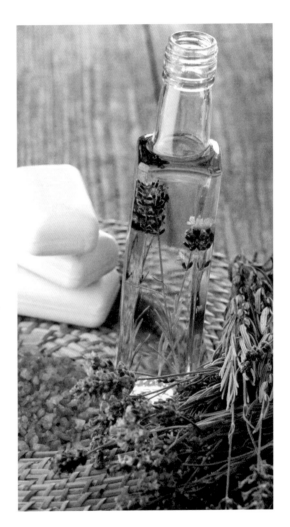

Properties of Oils

The oils and their actions are extremely complex. All the oils are antiseptic, but each one also has individual properties; for example, they may be analgesic, fungicidal, diuretic or expectorant. The collective components of each oil also work together to give it a dominant characteristic. It can be relaxing, refreshing or stimulating.

Essential oils also have notable physiological effects. Certain oils have an affinity with particular areas of the body. For example, rose has an affinity with the female reproductive system, while spice oils tend to benefit the digestive system. The oil may also sedate an overactive system, or stimulate a different part of the body that is sluggish. Some oils such as lavender are known as adaptogens, meaning they do whatever the body requires of them at the time. The psychological response is triggered by the effect of the aromatic molecules on the brain.

Treating Yourself

There are many ways to use essential oils at home. Massage and bathing tend to be the most popular, and techniques that involve applying oils to the body are usually more effective than inhalation. However, there are several other techniques that are particularly beneficial for certain conditions. These include steam inhalations, creams, lotions and shampoos, gargles and mouthwashes, neat applications (only appropriate for some oils), douches and compresses.

Carrier Oils

When essential oils are used for massage, they must be mixed into a base or carrier, as they are too concentrated and powerful to be used on the skin in an undiluted form. Carrier oils also provide the lubrication needed for the massage itself.

A carrier oil can be any unperfumed vegetable oil, such as soya, safflower or sunflower oils, although the oils most often used in aromatherapy are sweet almond oil and grapeseed oil. Some carrier oils have therapeutic qualities of their own – for example, peach kernel, avocado and apricot kernel are rich and nourishing, and high in vitamin E. Olive oil has many healing properties, although its strong odour sometimes masks the scent of the oil itself. A good ratio of oils is three drops of essential oil for every 5 ml of carrier oil.

Flowers

Flowers are used in essential oils for treating a wide range of ailments, from anxiety to throat infections. They were used as perfumes in ancient times to prevent diseases, then believed to be spread through bad odours. Their scents are among the most soothing of all oils, and flowers such as lavender have long been used to combat stress and aid sleep.

Rose *(Rosa centifolia, R. damascena)*

The rose has many therapeutic properties but its oil is very expensive to produce. The oil is distilled from the blossoms of the rose, usually from two types of roses, although there are many variations. The oils vary slightly in colour and fragrance, but have similar properties and uses. Rose oil can be used in tiny quantities and still be extremely effective.

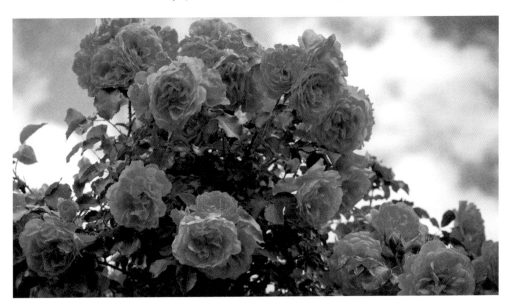

Female Ailments

A renowned aphrodisiac, sedative and a tonic with antidepressant properties, rose has an affinity with the female reproductive system, helping to regulate the menstrual cycle and alleviate premenstrual syndrome (PMS) or postnatal depression. Broken veins, ageing or wrinkled skin also benefit from treatment with the essential oil. Rose should not be used during the first three months of pregnancy and not at all if there is a history of miscarriage.

Other Uses

Rose is useful in treating headaches, earache, conjunctivitis, coughs and hay fever. In some cases it can help to encourage wound healing. Rose oil is a powerful antiseptic against viruses and bacteria; it acts as a tonic for the heart, circulation, liver, stomach and uterus, and helps to detoxify the blood and organs.

Jasmine *(Jasminum officinale)*

Jasmine is known as the king of essential oils, largely because it takes so many flowers to produce a small quantity of this expensive oil, and because just a little oil offers profound therapeutic benefits. Very rarely jasmine may cause an allergic reaction.

Help for Men and Women

Jasmine has a reputation as an aphrodisiac, reducing impotence in men and frigidity in women. It is also a uterine tonic which can help with period pain and disorders of the uterus; its pain-relieving properties and ability to strengthen contractions make it one of the best oils to use during childbirth; it is also believed to strengthen male sex organs and has been used for prostate problems. Its relaxing and antidepressant effect helps with postnatal depression.

Stress Relief

It is excellent for stress relief and is uplifting during times of lethargy. Jasmine has a soothing, warming and anti-inflammatory effect on joints and a rejuvenating effect on dry, wrinkled or ageing skin. Its antiseptic and expectorant properties also make it applicable for catarrh, chest and throat infections.

Lavender *(Lavandula angustifolia)*

Lavender has been used since ancient times for both its perfume and its medicinal qualities. Lavender is the most versatile and most widely therapeutic of all essential oils and has a huge range of therapeutic properties. Calming, soothing, antidepressant and emotionally balancing, its antiseptic, antibacterial and painkilling properties make it valuable in treating cuts, wounds, burns, bruises, spots, allergies, insect bites and throat infections. Lavender is the oil most associated with burns and healing of the skin, and can be applied neat to a burn to prevent infection and encourage speedy healing.

Breathe Easy

Because it is a decongestant it is also effective against colds, flu and catarrhal conditions. Lavender lowers blood pressure, prevents and eases digestive spasms, nausea and indigestion. It is antirheumatic and a tonic; problems of the nervous system such as tension, depression, insomnia, headaches, stress and hypertension all respond particularly well to its soothing properties.

A Word of Warning

Lavender is usually safe to use for all age groups, but some hay fever or asthma sufferers may be allergic to it. Lavandin is often sold as lavender because it is cheaper to produce, but be aware that it will not work.

Geranium *(Pelargonium graveolens)*

This lovely aromatherapy oil is traditionally regarded as a feminine oil, a powerful healer and a valuable insect repellent. Geranium is mentally uplifting and refreshing. It has a balancing effect on the nervous system, helping to alleviate apathy, anxiety, stress, hyper-activity and depression.

Anti-inflammatory and Antiseptic

The anti-inflammatory, soothing and astringent properties of geranium account for its success in treating arthritis, acne, nappy rash, burns, blisters, eczema, cuts and congested pores. Antiseptic properties make it useful for cuts and infections, sore throats and mouth ulcers. It is also a diuretic, used to relieve swollen breasts and fluid retention and to stimulate sluggish lymph and blood circulation.

Mind and Body in Balance

Geranium helps to stop bleeding and acts as a tonic for the liver and kidneys. It is used to treat PMS and menopausal problems and has a balancing effect on mind and body. Do not use geranium oil during the first three months of pregnancy, and not at all if there is a history of miscarriage.

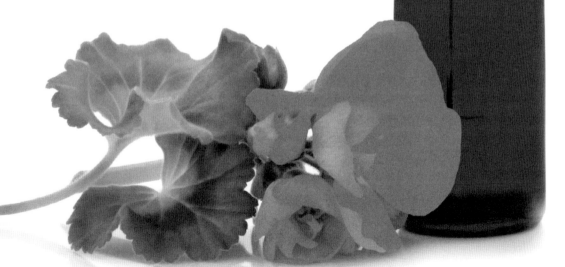

Plants

The flowers and leaves of many different plants can be distilled to extract their essential oils. With scents as mild as chamomile and as strong as peppermint, these oils can sooth and revitalize, offer pain relief and heal wounds.

Chamomile *(Chamaemelum nobile)*

Chamomile was sacred to the ancient Egyptians, who dedicated it to the Sun because it cured agues. It is one of the most gentle essential oils available, and particularly suitable for treating young children. Of the many varieties of chamomile available, Roman chamomile is one of the most commonly used in aromatherapy. Do not use in the first three months of pregnancy and refrain from using chamomile essential oil in the eyes.

Soothing Properties

Chamomile calms the nervous system and induces sleep. It has valuable anti-inflammatory, antiseptic and bactericidal properties. It prevents and eases spasms, relieves pain, settles digestion and acts as a liver tonic. Children with diarrhoea will respond to gentle massage of the abdomen with this oil and it can also be used to relieve headaches, toothache, period pain, arthritis and neuralgia. Indigestion, nausea and flatulence can also benefit and all manner of skin problems such as rashes, inflammation, cuts, boils, allergies, insect bites and chilblains can be helped by a chamomile compress; a few drops can be added to a warm bath to reduce weariness and ease pain in any part of the body.

Chamomile Inhalations

Inhalations will relieve the pain of headache, migraine, flu, coughs, facial neuralgia and sinusitis; massage a few drops in a light carrier oil around the nose and sinus area for almost immediate relief. It has a balancing effect on the menstrual cycle, reduces fluid retention and acts as a gentle antidepressant and stress reliever.

Peppermint
(Mentha piperita)

Peppermint is best known as a remedy for digestive problems. The essential oil is both a tonic and a stimulant, with a particular affinity for nervous

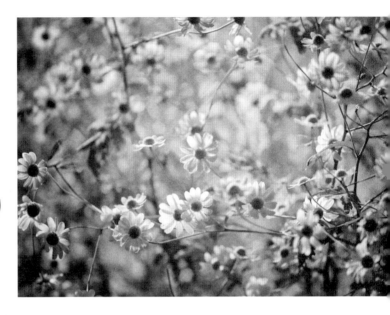

disorders, nervous vomiting, flatulence and colitis. Peppermint should not be used during pregnancy. Never use peppermint oil undiluted, as it can provoke a reaction. Also avoid using if you are taking homeopathic remedies, as it acts as an antidote.

Stomach Ailments

Refreshing and stimulating, peppermint tones and settles the digestive system – it relieves indigestion, flatulence, spasms, diarrhoea, nausea, stomach cramps and travel sickness; it also helps tone the stomach, liver, intestines and the nervous system. It is a valuable expectorant in the treatment of bronchitis, colds and flu, and it can reduce fevers by inducing sweating and cooling the body.

Pain Relief

Peppermint is a painkiller, beneficial for toothache, headaches and some migraines. It relieves itching, is a useful antiseptic for acne and congested skin, and is often used as an emergency remedy for shock. Muscle and mental fatigue are also relieved by peppermint.

Lemongrass *(Cymbopogon citrates)*

Lemongrass has been used in traditional Indian medicine for centuries. The essential oil is distilled from the grass leaves. It has a strong, refreshing citrus smell that has numerous aromatherapy and domestic uses. When using lemongrass, dilute it well as it may cause skin irritation in some people. Do not use on babies or children and do not use around the eyes.

Nerves and Muscles

Lemongrass has a tonic effect on the nervous system and the body in general. It can be used as a painkiller and antidepressant and is good for headaches, lethargy and symptoms of stress. It is also beneficial for muscular pain and poor muscle tone. It has fever-reducing properties and helps the immune system fight infections.

Deodorizing Properties

As a deodorant, lemongrass can be used for excessive perspiration and sweaty feet and its astringent properties make lemongrass an effective skin toner, which helps to close open pores. Lemongrass is also an effective flea, lice and tick repellent; use it in a vaporizer to keep flies out of the kitchen in summer and to get rid of pet smells from the home.

Melissa *(Melissa officinalis)*

Melissa, also known as heart's delight, has been used medicinally since the seventeenth century. The fresh lemony essential oil is distilled from the leaves and flowering tops. Dilute well as it may irritate some skin types.

Calming Effects

Melissa helps to reduce high blood pressure and, because it also helps to calm palpitations and rapid breathing, it is a good remedy for shock. Melissa calms the nervous system, relieves anxiety and has an uplifting effect on the emotions, dispelling sadness and loss, and counteracting hysteria. It also has a general tonic effect on mind and body.

All-round Benefits

The oil is often used for menstrual problems as it has a calming and regulating effect on the menstrual cycle, helps to ease period pain and improves missing or scanty periods. Melissa can be used to reduce digestive spasms in colic, nausea and indigestion, relieve migraine and combat fever. Low dilutions can be beneficial for eczema and other skin problems; allergies affecting the skin and the respiratory system can benefit from its antihistamine properties.

Juniper *(Juniperus communis)*

Physically and emotionally cleansing, juniper helps to detoxify the body of harmful waste products that contribute to problems such as rheumatoid arthritis and cellulite, and clears the mind of confusion and exhaustion. However, do not use juniper if pregnant or if you have a kidney disease.

Inside and Out

Juniper is also diuretic, has an affinity with the genitourinary system and is excellent for treating cystitis. Skin problems, especially weepy eczema and acne, also respond well to its toning, astringent and antiseptic properties. Juniper is good for haemorrhoids and hair loss, and assists with wound healing. It stimulates appetite, relieves nervous tension and is an excellent disinfectant.

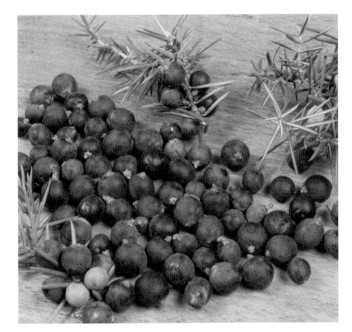

Trees

From precious sandalwood to refreshing pine, essential oils from trees around the world have been used to treat all manner of ailments for centuries. In ancient times, these oils were some of the most valued and revered of all traditional remedies.

Tea Tree *(Melaleuca alternifolia)*

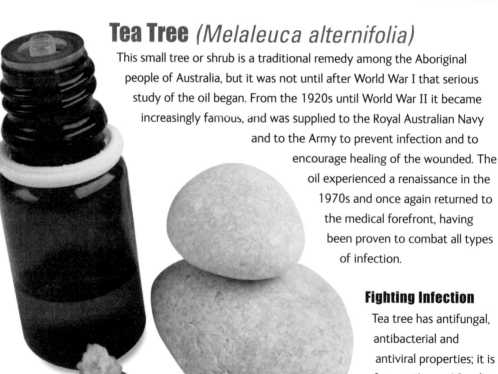

This small tree or shrub is a traditional remedy among the Aboriginal people of Australia, but it was not until after World War I that serious study of the oil began. From the 1920s until World War II it became increasingly famous, and was supplied to the Royal Australian Navy and to the Army to prevent infection and to encourage healing of the wounded. The oil experienced a renaissance in the 1970s and once again returned to the medical forefront, having been proven to combat all types of infection.

Fighting Infection

Tea tree has antifungal, antibacterial and antiviral properties; it is frequently used for skin problems such as spots, acne, warts, verrucae, athlete's foot, rashes, insect bites, burns and blisters, but it can be used to clean cuts and infected wounds and helps skin to heal by encouraging the formation of scar tissue. Tea tree can be used to treat cold sores and urinary or genital infections such as cystitis and thrush. However, people with sensitive skin should introduce the oil with caution.

Immune-system Stimulation

An expectorant that also alleviates inflammation and is a valuable immune stimulant, tea tree is known to boost the immune system, and is used in the treatment of colds, flu, respiratory infections, catarrhal problems and infectious illnesses; it is also used to reduce a fever. Tea tree is effective against dandruff and it is now a popular choice for delousing children's hair, providing effective treatment without the side-effects of drugs.

Sandalwood *(Santalum album)*

Sandalwood oil is one of the main remedies used in Ayurvedic (ancient Indian) medicine, and it is used to treat a wide variety of diseases. Its woody, sweet fragrance is often used in perfume and soap, particularly in Europe. The best sandalwood oil comes from India, where it is distilled from the mature tree.

Healing Properties

Sandalwood is an antiseptic, particularly effective for all urinary disorders, especially cystitis, probably because of its antibacterial properties. It clears catarrh and is effective for respiratory conditions such as bronchitis, dry coughs and sore throats. The oil helps to soothe the stomach, reduce digestive spasms, relieve fluid retention and reduce inflammation.

Soothing Skin

Sandalwood encourages wound healing and skin problems such as dry, chapped skin, acne, psoriasis, eczema and shaving rash can all benefit from its soothing, rehydrating and antiseptic action. It should not be used undiluted on the skin, however. It is an antidepressant oil that calms the nervous system. The oil is also considered to be somewhat aphrodisiac.

Pine *(Pinus sylvestris)*

The Arabs, Greeks and Romans all made use of the medicinal properties of the pine tree, while Native Americans are believed to have used pine to prevent scurvy and infestation with lice and fleas.

Refreshing and Stimulating

Inhalations of pine are wonderful for colds, catarrhal conditions including hay fever, and sore throats. The oil, which is expectorant, antiseptic and antiviral, helps to clear chest infections, sinuses and ease breathing. Pine stimulates the circulation and helps to relieve rheumatic and muscular aches, pains and stiffness. Pine is also deodorizing and insecticidal; it is good for excessive perspiration and to clear lice and scabies. Its refreshing aroma dispels apathy, relieves mental fatigue, nervous exhaustion and stress-related problems.

Advice on Using Pine Oil

Pine should only be used in small amounts in the bath or in massage. Do not use if you have an allergic skin condition. Always check the source of your oil as oils are distilled from several species of pine, some of which are unsuitable for use in aromatherapy.

Eucalyptus *(Eucalyptus globules)*

Several of the 700 species of eucalyptus are used to distil medicinal-quality essential oil, but the Australian 'blue gum' is by far the most widely used. Eucalyptus is a traditional remedy in Australia and a familiar ingredient in numerous chest rubs and decongestants. Do not take eucalyptus when using homeopathic remedies. Do not use for more than a few days at a time because of risk of toxicity. Do not use on babies or very young children.

Uses of Eucalyptus

Eucalyptus is used mostly for coughs, colds, chest infections and sinusitis. The oil is also used to reduce fevers and treat skin infections, cuts and blisters, genital and oral herpes, chicken pox and shingles. It alleviates inflammation generally and is helpful in treating rheumatism, muscular aches and pains and fibrositis. It is a diuretic and a deodorant, with strong antiviral and immune-stimulating properties and is an effective local painkiller, especially for nerve pain. Urinary tract problems such as cystitis respond well to regular use of the oil.

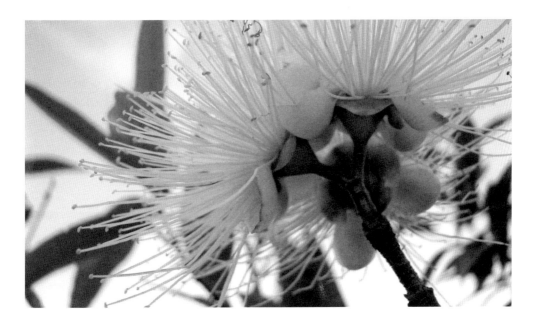

Ylang ylang *(Cananga odorata* var. *genuine)*

Ylang ylang is distilled from trees known as perfume trees, which originated in the Philippines and have now spread throughout Asia. The oil is distilled from the freshly picked flowers. The oil is very liquid, clear and has a heady fragrance with high notes of hyacinth and narcissus. Ylang ylang can cause nausea or headaches in high concentrations. It may also irritate some hypersensitive people.

Finding a Balance

Ylang ylang is an adaptogenic oil, which means that it can help to rebalance – working as either a stimulant or a relaxant. Sedative, antidepressant and a tonic for the nervous system, depression, anxiety, tension, irritability, and stress-related insomnia can all benefit from its soothing properties. It helps to rebalance sebum production in oily skin, acne and both dry and greasy scalps; it can also be used to calm irritated skin as well as bites and stings.

Effects on the Blood

Ylang ylang has also been attributed with aphrodisiac properties and can be used to treat sexual problems. It acts as a circulatory tonic and works to rebalance body functions generally; and it can help to reduce blood pressure and to slow breathing and heart rate in cases of shock or panic – experts recommend that people suffering from palpitations or low blood pressure should carry a small bottle of the oil to inhale when necessary.

Frankincense *(Boswellia sacra, B. frereana, B. bhaw-dajiana)*

Frankincense, also known as olibanum, is distilled from the resin produced by the bark of a small North African tree. Since ancient times it has been considered a spiritual oil, used by many to encourage meditation. Frankincense slows the breathing and calms the nervous and digestive systems, relieving anxiety, depression, nervous tension, emotional upsets and stress-related digestive problems.

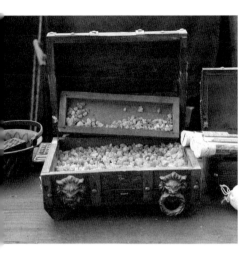

Practical Uses

As an immune stimulant and an expectorant, frankincense can help respiratory and catarrhal conditions such as asthma, colds, sinusitis, chest infections and chronic bronchitis. Frankincense has wound-healing, astringent, antiseptic and anti-inflammatory properties, making it ideal for treating cuts, scars, blemishes and inflammation, and it is recommended for firming ageing skin. Frankincense is helpful for cystitis as it has an affinity with the genitourinary system. Irregular or heavy periods and nosebleeds can also benefit from its healing properties.

Myrrh *(Commiphora myrrha)*

Perhaps best known as one of the three gifts brought to the infant Jesus, myrrh was valued in ancient times as an ingredient in embalming preparations, incense and as a medicine. Myrrh should not be used in high doses or at all during pregnancy.

The Oil of Kings

Myrrh has an excellent soothing, antiseptic and healing effect on sore or inflamed gums, mouth ulcers, wounds, and cracked or chapped skin. It can hasten the healing of weepy eczema and, because of its anti-fungal properties, it can be used as a vaginal wash for thrush or in a footbath for athlete's foot.

Myrrh is also an expectorant and a lung tonic, good for coughs, colds, bronchitis and flu. It stimulates, tones and soothes the digestive system and is often used for diarrhoea, haemorrhoids and indigestion. The oil acts as a uterine tonic, which can be helpful for menstrual irregularities. It relieves agitation, calms fears and uncertainties and has a positive, balancing effect on the emotions.

Fruits

The fruit, flowers and leaves of citrus trees provide some of the most refreshing and revitalizing essential oils. Used to combat everything from toxins in the body and cellulite to depression, fruit oils can clear the mind and purify the body.

Grapefruit Oil *(Citrus paradisi)*

Refreshing grapefruit oil is expressed from the peel of the fruit cultivated mainly in California, Brazil, Florida and Israel. It has a fresh, tangy, citrussy scent. Never ingest grapefruit oil orally and keep out of the eyes.

Flushing Out Toxins

As an antidepressant, grapefruit oil enlivens the mind, relieves anxiety and combats nervous exhaustion. Grapefruit is diuretic, detoxifying and cleansing to the kidneys; it also has a stimulating effect on the lymphatic system. Because of these properties it helps relieve fluid retention and eliminates the toxins that cause cellulite. It is also beneficial in a massage blend to ease stiff muscles after exercise. Grapefruit tones an oily skin and scalp, is helpful in treating acne and congested pores and can be applied neat to cold sores. It also stimulates digestion and improves immunity to infection.

Lemon *(Citrus limon)*

Lemons have been used for thousands of years for their therapeutic properties. The essential oil is obtained from the oily rind of the fruit. Lemon is refreshing and can help to ease the symptoms of depression. It can, however, irritate sensitive skin. Do not use before sunbathing, dilute well for massage and bath blends, and do not use for more than a few days at a time.

Fighting Infection

Lemon can stimulate the body's defences to fight all kinds of infection; it is beneficial in treating inflamed or diseased gums, mouth ulcers, sore throats and acne. It helps to clear colds, flu and bronchitis and can be used to remove warts and verrucae and to clear herpes blisters. The oil has a tonic effect on the circulation and is often used to treat varicose veins, poor circulation, high blood pressure and fluid retention.

Laxative and Astringent

Lemon is both a diuretic and a laxative and has the ability to stop bleeding in minor cuts and nosebleeds. As an astringent it benefits greasy skin and can also be used to reduce a fever; because it also counteracts acidity in the body, lemon helps to relieve acid indigestion, arthritis and rheumatism.

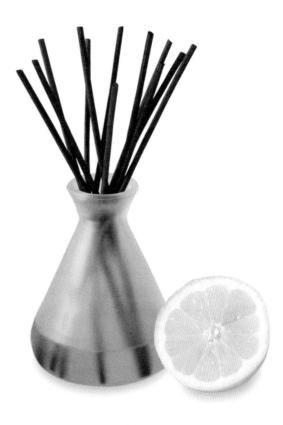

Bergamot *(Citrus aurantium var. bergamia)*

The bergamot tree was originally cultivated in Italy, where the fruit has a history of use in folk medicine. The refreshing essential oil is expressed from the peel of the fruit, which resembles a small yellow orange. Outside Italy bergamot is perhaps best known as an ingredient in both Earl Grey tea and eau de cologne. This bergamot is not to be confused with the herbs of the same name, *Monarda didyma* (also known as beebalm) and *Monarda fistulosa*, which are part of the mint family and are also used for medicinal, honey and ornamental purposes.

An Oil to Raise the Spirits

Joyous and uplifting, bergamot is a powerful antidepressant, which has a wonderful balancing effect on moods. As an antiseptic it is good for acne and boils, as well as other skin complaints such as oily skin, eczema and psoriasis; cuts and insect bites can often respond well. The oil inhibits viral activity and when diluted in alcohol, it can be dabbed on cold sores, chicken pox and shingles. Bergamot also has an affinity with the genitourinary system; it is a diuretic and a powerful urinary disinfectant, particularly good for cystitis; it can also be used for thrush and other types of vaginal itching and discharge. As a digestive, bergamot is sometimes used to encourage appetite; it is also used to cool fevers.

Advice on Using Bergamot

Bergamot increases the skin's sensitivity to sunlight. Never use it undiluted on the skin and simply avoid if you have sensitive skin. Mix it with a carrier oil before adding to bathwater to ensure it disperses well.

Neroli *(Citrus aurantium var. amara/bigaradia)*

The blossom of the bitter orange tree is used to produce this oil, which tones the heart and circulatory system. Its carminative (gas-preventing or relieving) and antispasmodic properties can relieve digestive problems such as indigestion, diarrhoea, flatulence and stomach cramps. Neroli helps to tone the skin and improve elasticity; added to cream or diluted in oil it is used to prevent stretch marks, scarring, wrinkles and to soothe sensitive skin. It is a gentle antidepressant and a nervous tonic, perhaps most helpful in treating anxiety, depression, nervous tension and stress-related problems. As a sedative it can also combat associated insomnia.

Petitgrain *(Citrus aurantium var. amara/bigaradia)*

Petitgrain is often regarded as a cheaper alternative to neroli. It is distilled from the leaves and twigs of the bitter orange tree, whereas neroli comes from the blossom. Petitgrain can refresh or relax, depending on the oils with which it is blended.

Stress Relief

It strengthens and tones the nervous system, and as such it can calm many stress-related problems such as nervous exhaustion and insomnia. Feelings of apathy, irritability, mild depression, anxiety, loneliness and pessimism can all get a lift from petitgrain's antidepressant properties. This oil also has a tonic effect during convalescence or when you are feeling run down; it has a notable antispasmodic effect and helps to tone the digestive system, relieving flatulence and indigestion.

Personal Hygiene

Petitgrain is a deodorant, sometimes used to control excessive perspiration; it is also used to control the overproduction of sebum in the skin and has gentle antiseptic properties, making it ideal for many greasy skin and scalp conditions, especially acne and greasy hair.

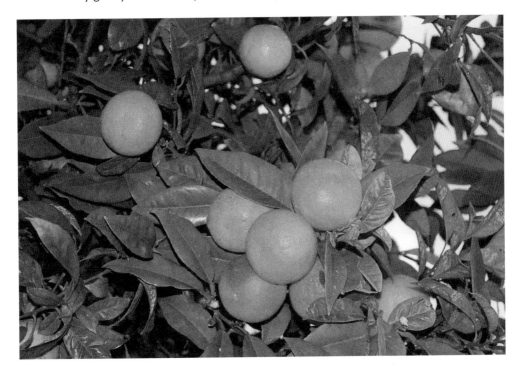

Herbs and Spices

Almost every part of herbal plants can be used in natural remedies, including the leaves, roots, seeds and flowers. Herbs and spices have been used for medicinal purposes – and in some religions were even considered sacred – since ancient times. Today, they are more popular than ever, for easing tired muscles, improving circulation, fighting infections and a multitude of other purposes.

Rosemary *(Rosmarinus officinalis)*

The word *Rosmarinus* means 'dew of the sea', and it relates to three species of evergreen flowering shrubs. Rosemary is one of the best-known and most used of the aromatic herbs. Rosemary oil tones the skin, liver and gall bladder; it is used to treat acne, eczema, dandruff, lice and hair loss. It also helps to clear catarrh, coughs and colds and headaches. It should not be used during pregnancy and is not suitable for people with epilepsy or high blood pressure.

A Herbal Tonic

Antiseptic and antibacterial, antifungal and a diuretic, generally cleansing and useful for fluid retention, Rosemary has properties that help to relieve painful periods and clear vaginal discharge, flatulence, indigestion and constipation. It works as a tonic for the nervous system and is an antidepressant; it relieves stress-related disorders, mental exhaustion and promotes mental clarity. A powerful circulation stimulant, excellent for low blood pressure, muscle fatigue, poor circulation, aches, pains and strains, it is both refreshing and rejuvenating, and acts as a perfect pick-me-up. Rosemary prevents and reduces digestive spasms, relieves wind and regulates digestion.

Hair Treatment

The oil is perhaps best-known for its effectiveness as a hair treatment; it is a tonic and conditioner of dark hair especially, helping to retain the colour; a little oil can be added to shampoos or rinses, and can help to reduce dandruff and prevent alopecia.

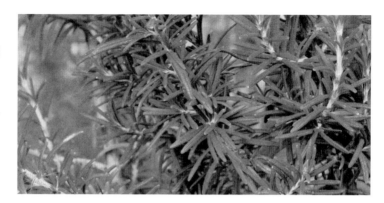

Sage *(Salvia officinalis)*

The properties of sage make this oil useful on its own or as part of a blend. It is effective in warming massages and acts as a general tonic for nervous and physical debility or where there are rheumatic pains. After a cold, use in the bath to warming effect. It has a softening effect on overworked muscles. Do not use in pregnancy, in feverish conditions, or in cases of high blood pressure.

Thyme *(Thymus vulgaris)*

One of the most useful medicinal herbs in natural health care, thyme was also one of the first plants to be used for its healing properties. The oil, distilled from the leaves and tiny purple flowering tops, has a fresh, green scent. Note when using thyme you should dilute it well, as it may cause irritation and sensitization in some people. Do not use if you have high blood pressure. It is best avoided during pregnancy and if you are taking homeopathic remedies.

Fighting Infection

Thyme is antiseptic and antibiotic, disinfectant and strongly germicidal; it is valuable for all infections especially gastric and bladder infections as it also has digestive and diuretic properties. Diluted oil is good for cleaning wounds, burns, bruises and clearing lice. It can also be used as a mouthwash as it helps to soothe and heal abscesses and gum infections.

Pain Relief

The oil's antirheumatic and antitoxic properties are beneficial in treating arthritis, gout and cellulite; rubefacient and stimulant actions help with muscle and joint pain and poor circulation. It stimulates the immune system to effectively fight off colds, flu and catarrh and ease coughing. Thyme has an uplifting fragrance, which can relieve depression, headaches and stress.

Marjoram *(Origanum majorana)*

In ancient times marjoram was reputed to promote longevity, a belief that encouraged the ancient Greeks to include it in perfumes, cosmetics and medicine. The essential oil is used to relieve agitation, dispel grief and restore calm, but should not be used during pregnancy.

Treating Muscle Aches

Marjoram is warming and pain relieving; it also has antispasmodic properties, making it good for muscle spasms and strains. It is a sedative and a nerve tonic which works to relieve nervous tension and promote restful sleep. Inhaling marjoram can help to relieve headaches and migraine.

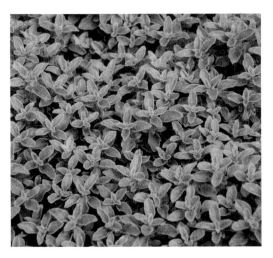

Everyday Ailments

Antiviral and bactericidal properties help to fend off colds and infections, and its expectorant properties make it a useful oil to include in a steam inhalation for chest infections. Massaged into the chest or throat, marjoram can also relieve painful coughs. The oil is a vasodilator, which is beneficial in treating high blood pressure and improving circulation. It also calms digestion, strengthens intestinal peristalsis and eases period pain.

Clary Sage *(Salvia sclarea)*

Also known as 'clear eye', clary sage was used in the Middle Ages for clearing foreign bodies from the eyes. It remains popular in aromatherapy because of its gentle action and pleasant fragrance. Do not use during pregnancy or when drinking alcohol as it can intoxicate, cause drowsiness and nightmares.

Lifting Spirits

Clary sage is an antidepressant and is sometimes described as a euphoric. It helps to regulate the nervous system and can help to prevent and arrest convulsion. It is most beneficial in treating anxiety, depression and stress-related problems. Clary sage is often recommended for absent or scanty periods and PMS, and is an aphrodisiac that can alleviate lack of sex drive and impotence.

Other Uses

It acts as a powerful muscle relaxant, helps ease muscular aches and pains and benefits digestion, relieves indigestion and flatulence. Its astringent properties make it useful for oily skin and scalp conditions. It is antibacterial and useful for throat and respiratory infections.

Fennel Oil *(Foeniculum vulgare)*

In folklore, fennel was believed to convey courage and strength and contribute to a long life. It also has a history of use as an antidote to poisons. When using fennel in aromatherapy, make sure you use only sweet fennel (also known as Roman or French fennel), as bitter fennel should not be used on the skin. Do not use during pregnancy. It is not suitable for epileptics or children under the age of six and is a narcotic in large doses.

Hormones in Harmony

Fennel appears to have a rebalancing effect on hormones, probably due to an oestrogenic-like plant hormone. It is a good diuretic, antimicrobial and antiseptic, which can help with premenstrual water retention and urinary tract infections. It helps to eliminate toxic wastes from the body, making it valuable in treating arthritis and cellulite.

Digestive and Other Benefits

It reduces digestive spasms, calms and tones the stomach and digestive system and has a slightly laxative effect, benefiting nausea, indigestion, constipation and stomach cramps. Fennel makes a good mouthwash for gum disease or infections.

Patchouli *(Pogostemon cablin)*

Patchouli is the aromatic oil extracted from a south-east Asian shrub of the mint family. It has many uses, and is especially pleasant when used as part of a blend. An important antidepressant, nervous tonic and reputed to be an aphrodisiac, patchouli is valued in treating depression, anxiety, nervous exhaustion, stress-related problems and lack of interest in sex. It is astringent, antiviral, antiseptic and anti-inflammatory, good for cracked skin and open pores; it is also effective for acne, eczema and dermatitis. Its fungicidal and deodorant actions make it one of the best choices for treating dandruff and fungal infections on the skin. It is a cell regenerator, good for ageing skins and promoting wound healing. It also acts as a diuretic.

Hyssop *(Hyssopus officinalis)*

Revered as a sacred cleansing herb by the Hebrews and the ancient Greeks, hyssop has also long been valued by herbalists for its medicinal properties. Both the leaves and the small blue or mauve flowers are distilled for their essential oil. Dilute well and use for no more than a few days at a time, because there is some risk of toxicity. Do not use during pregnancy or if you are epileptic. For people with high blood pressure, hyssop should only be used by a qualified aromatherapist.

Colds, Cuts and Circulation

Hyssop is an expectorant with antispasmodic, bactericidal and antiseptic properties, which can be helpful for coughing, whooping cough, catarrh, sore throats and chest infections. It can be used in skincare for cuts, bruises and inflammation. Hyssop has hypertensive properties making it useful in the treatment of low blood pressure and it has a general tonic effect on circulation.

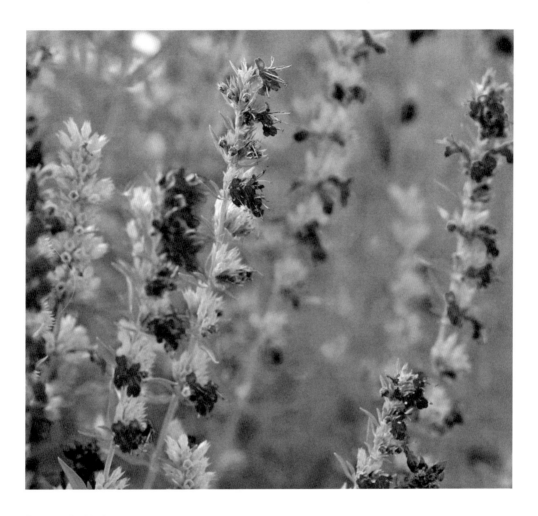

Stress Relief

As an emmenagogue (a herb that can stimulate blood flow in the pelvic and uterine area, and thus encourage menstruation), hyssop can be used for scanty or missing periods; the oil can also soothe indigestion and relieve colicky cramps. Hyssop's sedative and tonic properties can benefit stress or anxiety-related problems; it helps to clarify thinking, relieve fatigue and increase alertness.

Cinnamon *(Cinnamomum zeylanicum)*

The best cinnamon oil is believed to come from Madagascar. The medicinal properties of cinnamon were valued by the ancients and according to legend, it can have the effect of enhancing psychic ability and can act as an aphrodisiac. Cinnamon-leaf oil may cause skin irritation. Use only in a one per cent dilution and in moderation. Do not confuse with cinnamon bark oil, which is an irritant and should not be used in aromatherapy.

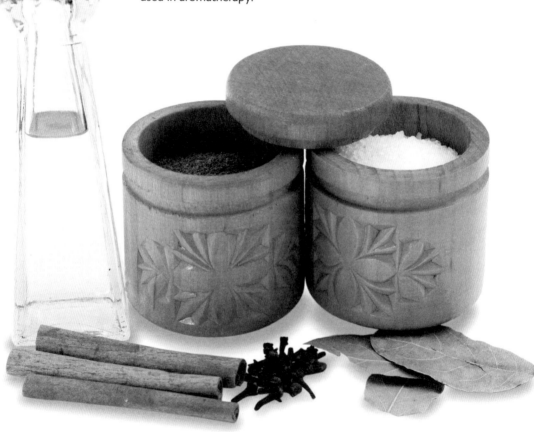

Stimulatory and Antiseptic Effects

Cinnamon stimulates a sluggish digestion, relieves flatulence and spasms and combats intestinal infection. It also stimulates respiration and circulation, helping with rheumatic problems and chest infections. It can help fortify the immune system against chills and infections and has a cooling effect on fevers. Cinnamon also has antiseptic, anti-microbial and parasiticidal properties, making it good for head lice, scabies and other skin infections. Cinnamon can relieve mental fatigue, improve concentration and nervous exhaustion and help lift depression.

Cloves *(Eugenia caryophyllata)*

This pungent, aromatic and warming herb helps to calm the digestive tract, soothing wind and easing nausea. It is beneficial to the lungs and is useful for people who feel cold and are prone to colds. Use clove oil sparingly and only when combined with a carrier oil before use. It can irritate or burn the skin when used directly. It has diverse uses, including as an insect repellent and an air freshener. As an antiseptic it can be used locally on swellings and for pains in the gums and teeth. Used sparingly in a bath it can help to ease confusion and lethargy.

Home Remedies

Cloves can be used as a home remedy for several ailments.

- **Abscess**: Oil of cloves can be chewed or placed directly on a sore tooth or mouth abscess to draw out the infection.

- **Fevers and vomiting**: Clove tea is a warming drink that can encourage the body to sweat, which is helpful in cases of high fever or vomiting.

- **Stomach acid**: Steep cloves in boiling water, simmer, strain and use the remaining liquid as a mild sedative and to soothe an acid stomach.

- **Wind**: Clove tea can be used to soothe wind and ease nausea, particularly travel sickness.

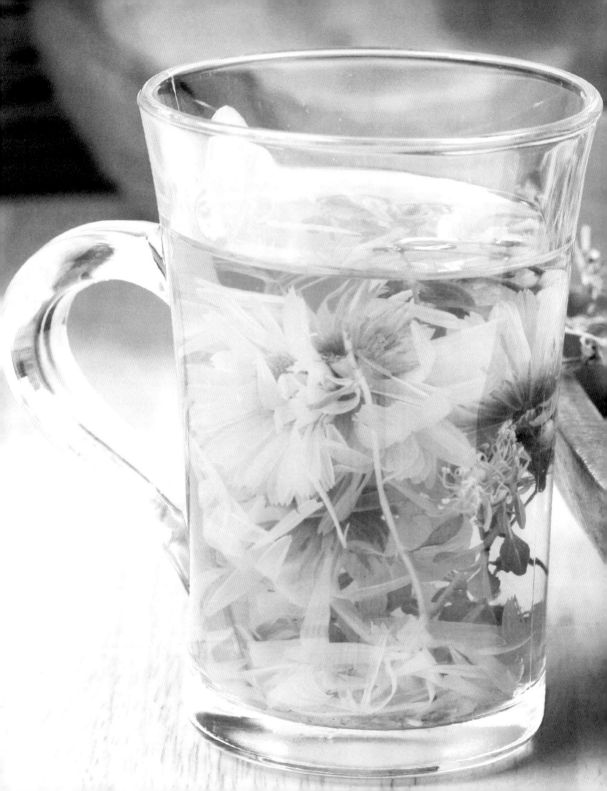

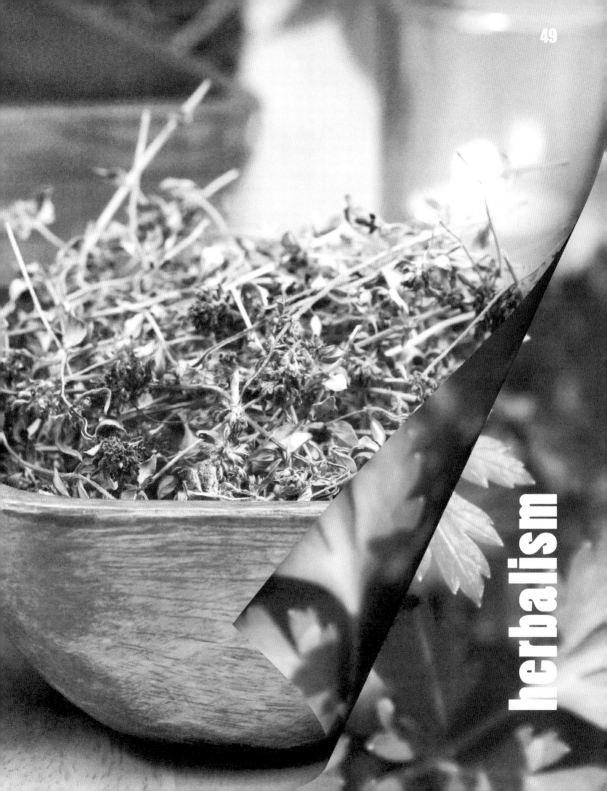

herbalism

Understanding Herbalism

Herbalism embraces the use of plants, in particular herbs, for healing. While herbs are used in many cultures – most specifically China and India – the tradition of Western medical herbalism is a rich and varied one, calling upon folk remedies, ancient customs and practical experience, and combined with new research, clinical training and diagnostic skills.

Herbal Healing

Herbal medicine is based on a holistic approach to health, like many other complementary medicines, and treatment will be undertaken after an assessment of your individual symptoms as well as your lifestyle and overall health, on both a physical and spiritual level.

Advice and treatment are always tailored to individual needs and because of this there is far less chance of having an adverse reaction to treatment. The aim of herbalism is to help the body heal itself and to restore balanced health, not just to relieve the symptoms of the disorder being treated.

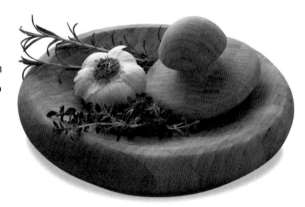

All-round Health

Herbalism is not a miracle cure and, like any other therapy, works best for specific conditions. Having said that, almost anyone can benefit from the prudent use of herbs as a form of restorative and preventative medicine. Herbs are a rich source of vitamins and minerals, aside from having healing properties, and can be an important part of your daily diet, eaten fresh, or perhaps drunk as a tisane.

Common Conditions

Some of the most common conditions that respond to herbal treatment include: hay fever, colds and respiratory disorders, digestive disorders (like constipation and ulcers), cardiovascular disease, headaches, anxiety, depression, chronic infections, rheumatism, arthritis, skin problems, anaemia and many hormonal, menstrual, menopausal and pregnancy problems.

A Summary of Herbs

A herb is any part of a flower, tree or other plant. Herbage, like foliage, refers to plants with green leaves but in herbal remedies more than leaves are used. Any part of a plant can be used, for example:

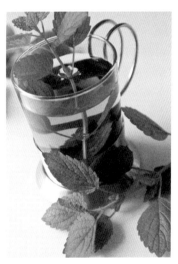

- **Flowers**: chamomile, marigold, linden, St John's wort
- **Leaves**: peppermint, sage, thyme, comfrey
- **Bark**: willow, oak, cinnamon
- **Buds**: cloves
- **Seeds**: fennel, cardamom
- **Fruits**: cayenne, rose hips
- **Root**: dandelion, marshmallow
- **Inner sap or gel**: aloe
- **Bulb**: garlic
- **Wood**: pau d'arco
- **Resin**: myrrh, frankincense

How Herbs Work

The chemical make-up of plants is extraordinarily complicated, with each element having specific roles within the body outside the active ingredient itself. For example, aspirin – one of the most common drugs to be related to the active ingredient of a plant (in this case white willow) – is very irritating to the stomach, often causing bleeding and gastric ulcers.

Meadowsweet, another herb with aspirin-like components, has anti-inflammatory as well as analgesic properties. In fact, it is often used to soothe damaged digestive systems, reducing the acidity of the stomach. The actions of the herbs are widespread within the body, not just addressing the condition at hand, but increasing vitality and replacing deficiencies that could cause problems in the future.

Herbalism in Practice

There are a number of ways in which herbalism is applied practically. A herbal tonic is useful, for example, in the winter months when fresh fruit and green vegetables are not a regular part of our diets. Echinacea or garlic, for instance, can be taken daily to improve the general efficiency of the immune system. They can be applied externally as compresses or made into tinctures.

Infusions

Effectively another word for tea, an infusion uses dried herbs, or in some instances fresh, which are steeped in boiled water for about 10 minutes. Infusions are most suitable for plants from which the leaves and flowers are used, since their properties are more easily extracted by gentle boiling. Tisanes are mild infusions, usually pre-packaged and sold in the form of a teabag, which can be boiled for a much shorter period of time than an infusion.

Decoctions

The roots, twigs, berries, seeds and barks of a plant are used to make a decoction – they are boiled in water to extract the plants' ingredients. The liquid is strained and taken with a bit of honey or brown sugar as prescribed. Decoctions should be refrigerated and will last about three days.

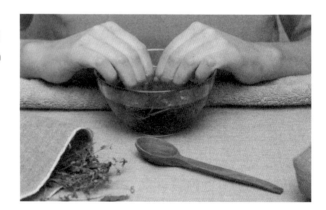

Tinctures

Tinctures are one of the most powerful and concentrated forms of herbal medicine. Powdered, fresh or dried herbs are placed in an airtight container with alcohol and left for a period of time. Alcohol extracts the valuable or essential parts of the plant and preserves them for the longest possible time. You can make your own tincture at home. Dosages are usually 5–20 drops, which can be taken directly or added to water.

Gargles

Many herbs can be prepared in the form of a gargle, which has the same therapeutic benefits as an essential-oil gargle. Simply use an infusion, decoction or mix a few drops of tincture in cooled, boiled water and gargle. Most herbs can be safely swallowed. Dilute four to five drops of essential oil in a teaspoon of brandy. Mix into a glass of warm water and swish around the mouth or use as a gargle. Do not swallow.

Compresses and Poultices

Compresses and poultices are for external use and can be extremely effective, since the active parts of the herb are able to reach the affected area without being altered by the digestive tract in any way.

 Poultice: A poultice is made up of a plant which has been crushed and then applied whole to the affected areas. You can also boil crushed plant parts for a few minutes to make a pulp, which will act as a poultice, or use a powdered herb and mix with boiling water. Because they are most often applied with heat and use fresh parts of the plant, they are usually more potent than compresses.

 Compresses: These are usually made from infusions or decoctions which are used to soak a linen or muslin cloth. The cloth is then placed on the affected area, where it can be held in place by a bandage or plastic wrap. Compresses can be hot or cold and are generally milder than poultices.

Flowers

Flowers such as echinacea and St John's wort have recently become staples of the medicine cabinet in many homes – their healing properties widely acknowledged. Flowers are used by herbalists to treat ailments as diverse as depression and heartburn, as many have a calming effect on the mind and body.

Echinacea
(Echinacea angustifolia and *E. purpurea)*

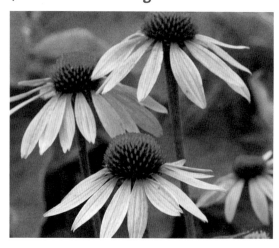

Echinacea is known as the purple cone flower, and is native to North America. It has become a bastion of natural health care, with its powerful and now well-proven ability to improve immunity. One of the primary remedies for helping the body rid itself of microbial infections, it is often effective against both bacterial and viral attacks, and may be used in conditions such as boils, septicaemia and similar infections.

Echinacea activates the body to destroy both cancerous cells and pathogens, increases the level of white blood cells and boosts the immune system in general. It is especially useful for infections of the upper respiratory tract such as laryngitis, tonsillitis and for catarrhal conditions of the nose and sinus. It may be used as an external lotion to help septic sores and cuts.

Tips for Taking Echinacea

Echinacea is often – inappropriately – used as a daily immune-system support. Daily intake should only take place during the cold and flu season but for chronic infections such as chronic hepatitis, echinacea may be used continuously for several months. However, for the maintenance of a healthy immune system echinacea is most wisely used periodically – a few weeks on, and a few weeks off, throughout the year.

Echinacea Decoction

To make a decoction, put one to two teaspoonfuls of the root in one cup of water and bring it slowly to boil. Let it simmer for 10–15 minutes. This should be drunk three times a day. Take 1–4 ml of the tincture three times a day.

St John's Wort *(Hypericum perforatum)*

St John's wort has become one of the most popular antidepressant herbs, and recent studies show that it is as effective, if not more so, than the drug Prozac. It does, however, have a wide variety of other therapeutic uses. It strengthens and speeds healing in the nervous system, is analgesic, antiviral and anti-inflammatory. It treats neuralgia, sciatica, pain with tingling in hands or feet and back pain. St John's wort can be used internally and externally for pain from deep wounds.

Effects of Oils and Tinctures

Use as a tincture as lotion for shingles, cold sores and herpes. Use as a cream for sore skin, inflamed rashes and cuts. Use infused oil as a base oil for aromatherapy back massage and with lavender essential oil for neuralgia.

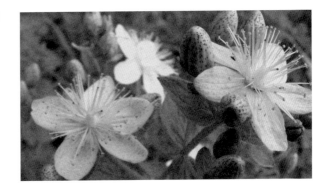

Long-term Use

Note that it may be a week before depression begins to lift. The best preparations for external use are the infused oil and creams based on the infused oil. For nerve damage you may need to persist for some months. Do not take with prescription drugs, unless on the advice of a registered herbalist.

Rose *(Rosa damascena)*

Rose oil is normally used therapeutically, but red roses may also be used as a herb. They can be a valuable tonic for the heart and lungs. As a tea, the petals are astringent and have a tonic effect on the gut and liver.

Herbal Uses for Rose

Rose has a diuretic action and is said to increase appetite. It can have a soothing effect on the skin. Rose petals are a good addition to any herbal remedy when there are emotional aspects, particularly a feeling of 'holding back'. Use in a tea, in gentle creams for the skin and in the bath.

Lavender *(Lavandula angustifolia)*

This fragrant herb has a wide range of uses. As an infusion and a tea it acts by carrying blood away from the head and relaxes the nervous system, making it good for pains, cramps and burns. It can also be helpful for insomnia and tension headaches. It is antiseptic and therefore useful for urinary tract infections. Lavender has a soothing, cleansing effect on delicate skin and is good as an infusion for washing the face and hair.

Lavender Infusions

Infuse one teaspoon of the herb in a cup of boiling water and drink three times a day. Or dilute 1–2 ml of tincture in water and take three times a day.

Calendula *(Calendula officinalis)*

Also known as marigold, the whole flower tops or petals of the common garden plant are used therapeutically. Calendula is one of the best herbs for treating local skin problems. It also has a marked antifungal activity and may be used both internally and externally. It can be used safely wherever there is an inflammation on the skin, whether due to infection or physical damage. Calendula may be used for any external bleeding or wounds, bruising or strains. It will also be of benefit in slow-healing wounds and skin ulcers. It is ideal for first-aid treatment of minor burns and scalds.

Properties and Uses

Calendula has many valuable properties and uses.

- **Properties**: Anti-inflammatory, antispasmodic, lymphatic, astringent, emmenagogue, antimicrobial.

- **Internally**: Acts as a valuable herb for digestive inflammation and thus it may be used in the treatment of gastric and duodenal ulcers.

- **Cholagogue**: Will aid the relief of gall-bladder problems and also through this processs aid digestion.

- **Antifungal**: Has marked antifungal activity and may be used internally and externally.

Yarrow *(Achillea millefolium)*

Yarrow is a sacred plant to many cultures. In China, yarrow stalks were used to cast the I Ching, to read the future for the emperor. Ayurvedics use the herb as a 'heal-all' because it has so many uses – allowing you to keep your head in the heavens and your feet on the ground. Yarrow balances emotional upsets, and is a frequent addition to treatments during menopause.

Uses for Yarrow

Yarrow can be used for the early stages of fevers, especially with hot, dry skin. It treats catarrh, sinusitis, hay fever and dust allergies and is useful in high blood pressure, with hawthorn and linden. Use it with a little ginger for cold feet. Yarrow can be used internally and externally for varicose veins and spontaneous bruising, for thrombosis and to prevent blood clots; apply the infused oil to inflammations associated with varicose veins.

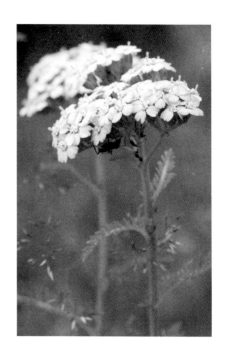

Vervain *(Verbena officinalis)*

This herb Is good for anxiety and is often given for anxious states during pregnancy because of its high iron content. Use it as a tonic, fever herb, nerve restorative, antispasmodic, carminative or diuretic. It alleviates exhaustion, post-viral fatigue and exhaustion from overwork or nervous depression. Vervain also treats fevers and flu, especially with headaches and nervous symptoms, including insomnia, excessive dreaming and feelings of paranoia.

General Tonic Effects

Vervain is a good general tonic, relieving many problems: indigestion, worms and parasites, digestive discomfort following treatment for parasites, liverishness with nausea, heavy headaches and depression, irritable bowel syndrome with mucus in the stools, asthma, period pains, post-operative tiredness and depression.

Using Vervain

Sip the tea throughout labour to encourage regular contractions; continue after the birth to encourage milk flow; it also treats postnatal depression. Standard-strength teas should be taken every two hours in fevers or three cups a day for chronic complaints. For worms and parasites make double-strength tea and drink before breakfast.

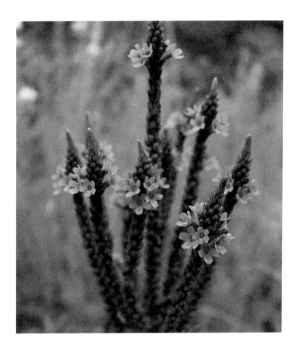

Chamomile
(Chamomilla recutita)

This is a wild plant with small, daisy-like flowers. Chamomile is a very safe herb, especially suitable for children, and can be taken freely. It can cause an allergic rash but this disappears on stopping usage.

Properties and Uses

Chamomile is calming and soothing with anti-inflammatory, antiseptic, antispasmodic and digestive properties. It can help anxiety, tension, headaches and insomnia, and any kind of digestive upset including acidity, heartburn, wind and colic. The lotion or cream is good for itchy skin conditions. It is also good for restless and over-excitable children and most children's complaints including fevers and teething troubles; chamomile is especially helpful for infants. Although chamomile is sold in tea bags as a herbal drink for everyday use, it should not be overlooked as a medicinal herb; it is gentle but very powerful.

Feverfew *(Tanacetum parthenium)*

Feverfew is a small-flowered daisy, easily grown in gardens and window boxes. Use it as an anti-inflammatory, antispasmodic and emmenagogue. It can relieve migraine and arthritis; use it with valerian for migraine linked with anxiety and tension.

Feverfew Tinctures

The best preparation is the tincture made from the fresh plant. Use one teaspoon in a little water at the first signs of a migraine, repeat in two hours if necessary. For repeated attacks and as a treatment for arthritis take one teaspoon every morning. If you have a plant, two or three medium-sized leaves equals one teaspoon of tincture.

Elderflower *(Sambucus nigra)*

Elderflower is a popular herb in natural remedies and is one of the main diaphoretic herbs (it encourages perspiration and the elimination of toxins). Elderflowers and elderberries are nutritious and work as a laxative among other things. Different parts of the plant are used:

- **Bark**: Used therapeutically as a purgative, emetic and diuretic.

- **Leaves**: Used externally as an emollient and internally as a purgative, expectorant, diuretic and diaphoretic.

- **Flowers**: Diaphoretic, anticatarrhal and antispasmodic.

- **Berries**: Diaphoretic, diuretic and laxative.

Different Parts for Different Ailments

The elder tree is a medicine chest in itself. The leaves are used for bruises, sprains, wounds and chilblains. It has been reported that elder leaves may be useful in an ointment for tumours. Elderflowers are ideal for the treatment of colds and flu. They are indicated as being useful against any catarrhal inflammation of the upper respiratory tract such as hay fever and sinusitis. Catarrhal deafness too responds well to elderflowers. Elderberries have similar properties to the flowers with the addition of their usefulness in rheumatism.

Preparing an Infusion

Pour one cup of boiling water on to two teaspoonfuls of the dried or fresh blossoms and infuse for 10 minutes. Drink hot three times a day. To make a juice, boil fresh berries in water for two to three minutes, then express the juice. To preserve, bring to the boil with one part honey to 10 parts of juice. Take one glass diluted with hot water twice a day. For the ointment, take three parts of fresh elder leaves and heat them with six parts of melted Vaseline until the leaves are crisp. Strain and store. The tincture (made from the flowers) should be taken 2–4 ml three times a day.

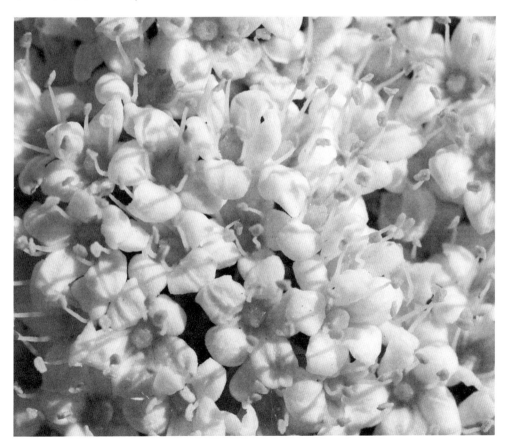

Fruits and Berries

The fruits and berries of different plants contain much of the goodness. As well as vital vitamins, fruits used in herbalism have many other beneficial properties when consumed directly or made into a tincture.

Bilberry *(Vaccinium myrtillus)*

Also known as blueberry, the bilberry is a strong antioxidant that keeps capillary walls strong and flexible. It also helps to maintain the flexibility of the walls of the red blood cells and allows them to pass through the capillaries better. The entire plant is used in treatment. Bilberry contains fatty acids, flavonoids, iron, tannins and ursolic acid. It can also interfere with iron absorption when taken regularly.

Properties and Uses

These small berries contain a wealth of beneficial properties that can treat a variety of ailments:

- Helps control insulin levels
- Strengthens connective tissues

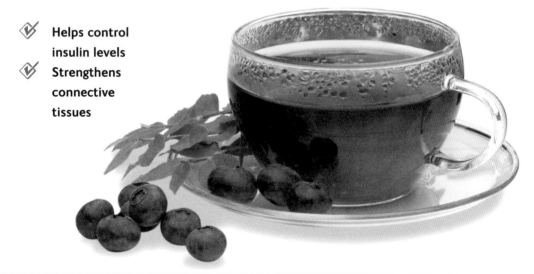

Inhibits the growth of bacteria

 Acts as an anti-inflammatory

 Anti-ageing and anti-carcinogenic

 Acts as a diuretic and urinary tract antiseptic

 Useful for hypoglycaemia and inflammation

 Can treat stress, anxiety, night blindness and cataracts

May help to halt or prevent macular degeneration

Agnus Castus *(Vitex agnus-castus)*

The fruit of a pretty Mediterranean shrub, half-hardy in the UK, balances hormones and relieves pre-menstrual syndrome with irritability, breast pain and water retention. It also helps menopausal symptoms, especially mood swings and depression. It can be taken with sage to treat hot flushes. It can restore a regular menstrual cycle when coming off the contraceptive pill or when the cycle has been disrupted.

Taking Agnus Castus

The best time to take these berries is first thing in the morning, before breakfast. One cup of the decoction, or 20–30 drops of the tincture in a little water, daily, will usually suffice.

Juniper *(Juniperus communis)*

The berries of this popular plant are most often used in herbalism. They contain a variety of therapeutic properties, including essential oils, but may interfere with the absorption of iron and other minerals when taken internally.

Herbal Uses of Juniper

Juniper acts as a diuretic, helps to regulate blood-sugar levels and relieves inflammation and congestion. It can be helpful in the treatment of asthma, bladder infection, fluid retention, gout, kidney problems, obesity and prostate disorders.

Leaves

From common garden herbs such as sage and thyme to traditional eastern shrubs, the leaves of many different plants are used in herbalism, often taken as infusions or drunk as teas.

Raspberry *(Rubus idaeus)*

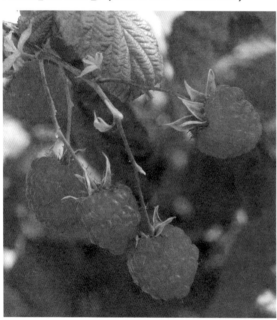

The leaves of the common raspberry plant are used in herbal medicine, and they have a long tradition of use during pregnancy. Raspberry leaves strengthen and tone the tissue of the womb, assisting contractions and checking any haemorrhage during labour. As an astringent raspberry may be used in a wide range of cases, including diarrhoea, leucorrhoea and other loose conditions. It is valuable in the easing of mouth problems such as mouth ulcers, bleeding gums and inflammations; as a gargle it will help sore throats. Raspberry is also very rich in iron and calcium.

Raspberry Infusions

For an infusion, pour a cup of boiling water on to two teaspoonfuls of the dried herb and let it infuse for 10–15 minutes. This may be drunk freely. Take 2–4 ml of the tincture three times a day. Do not take during the first three months of pregnancy, unless under medical supervision.

Peppermint *(Mentha piperita)*

One of the most popular herb teas in the world, peppermint is easily grown in the garden. It is digestive, carminative, antispasmodic, a mild stimulant and an emmenagogue. Peppermint can be taken freely. A small amount of peppermint may be added to most herb teas for flavour.

Common Ailments

It is used to treat indigestion, colic, wind, nausea, vomiting, depressed appetite, period pains and gall-bladder pain. A couple of drops of the essential oil in hot water, or sucking a strong peppermint sweet is also effective. Use with elderflower and yarrow for colds, sinus problems and blocked nose. A strong tea, used as a lotion, is good for hot, itchy skin problems.

Lemon Balm *(Melissa officinalis)*

A common plant in Britain, Europe, Western Asia and North Africa, lemon balm (also called balm or melissa) is used fresh, if in season, or the leaves can be dried for remedies. Its properties include:

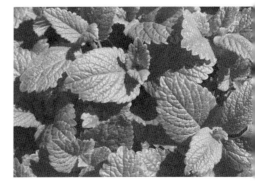

- ✔ **Carminative**
- ✔ **Nervine (beneficial for the nervous system)**
- ✔ **Antispasmodic**
- ✔ **Antidepressive**
- ✔ **Diaphoretic**
- ✔ **Antimicrobial**
- ✔ **Hepatic (beneficial for the liver)**

Uses

The balm is an excellent carminative herb that relieves spasms in the digestive tract and is used in flatulent dyspepsia; because of its mild antidepressive properties, it is primarily used where there is dyspepsia associated with anxiety or depression, as the gently sedative oils relieve tension and stress reactions, thus acting to lighten depression. It may be used for migraines that are associated with tension, neuralgia, anxiety-induced palpitations and insomnia. Lemon balm has a tonic effect on the heart and circulatory system which can lower blood pressure. It can be used in feverish conditions such as flu.

Infusing Lemon Balm

For an infusion, pour a cup of boiling water on to two or three teaspoonfuls of the dried herb or four to six fresh leaves and leave to infuse for 10–15 minutes, well covered until drunk. A cup of this tea should be taken in the morning and the evening, or when needed. Take the tincture 2–6 ml three times a day.

Parsley *(Petroselinum crispum)*

Native to the eastern Mediterranean, this popular herb is cultivated worldwide. Parsley can be used as a diuretic, expectorant, emmenagogue, carminative, antispasmodic and hypotensive remedy. The essential oil is obtained from the leaves and the seeds, and is used in aromatherapy. Do not use during pregnancy in medicinal dosage.

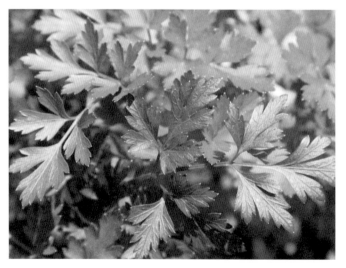

Tonic Effects

Parsley is a tonic in its effect on the blood vessels and is sometimes used in the treatment of haemorrhoids. Applied as a compress to bruises, parsley helps to shrink the broken blood vessels below the skin. The principle action of parsley is as a diuretic, and it is used in the treatment of urinary tract problems.

Sage *(Salvia officinalis)*

The actions of red sage and sage are very similar and can be used to treat any inflamed and septic mouth conditions. Sage is an astringent, a stimulant, antiseptic, carminative, antispasmodic, nervine and is generally strengthening. It alleviates depression and nervous exhaustion, post-viral fatigue and general debility.

It is good to treat anxiety and confusion in elderly people or accompanying exhaustion and weakened states. It soothes indigestion, wind, loss of appetite and mucus on the stomach. Do not use in pregnancy.

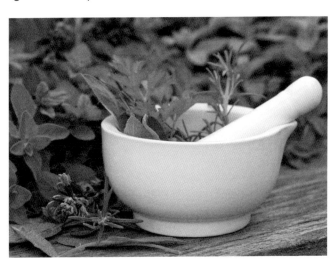

Other Benefits

Sage can alleviate the pressures of weak lungs with persistent and recurrent coughs and allergies. As a tea and a compress it is good for menopausal hot flushes, period pains and pre-menstrual painful breasts. Cold sage tea taken every few hours will usually dry up breast milk. It can also be used as a gargle and mouthwash for sore throats, laryngitis, tonsillitis, mouth ulcers and inflamed and tender gums, and as an antiseptic wash for dirty and slow-to-heal wounds.

Teas, Tinctures and Gargles

Traditionally, one cup a day maintains health in old age. For an extra-strength gargle add five drops of tincture of myrrh (from chemists or herb shops) to a cup of sage tea. Sage tincture can be taken, instead of the cold tea, for stopping night sweats: four teaspoons daily, in a little water.

Thyme *(Thymus vulgaris)*

This herb is popular in cooking. There are many different garden varieties with distinctive foliage: white thyme, yellow thyme, variegated thyme. Although not as strong as common wild *Thymus vulgaris*, they can be used in all recipes if nothing else is available.

Properties and Uses

Thyme is antiseptic, antibacterial, antifungal, expectorant and a digestive tonic. It can be used for whooping cough and any cough with infected or tough phlegm; it can be helpful, if taken regularly, in asthma. Thyme relieves indigestion, wind and intestinal infections. Use it with marshmallow for cystitis. It can cure intestinal worms in children and even, in a weak tea, to prevent nightmares. Thyme vinegar is antifungal for athlete's foot; dilute with an equal amount of water for washes and douches for thrush.

Dosage

Thyme can be taken freely and large doses might be needed for coughs. For an infant's coughs use two or three teaspoons of syrup up to four times daily. Make a chest rub from the infused oil. For children's worms, use quarter to half a cup of strong tea before breakfast, for two weeks.

Rosemary *(Rosmarinus officinalis)*

Rosemary has many traditional uses and stories. Most uses are based on elements of truth. Ophelia gave Hamlet a sprig for remembrance. It is planted in cemeteries for the same reason and it does help improve the memory by improving the circulation. During the Plague in Europe, posies of herbs, including rosemary, were carried to ward off the disease.

Restorative Effects

Rosemary lifts the spirits and improves circulation; it can also alleviate depression. It can help with headaches associated with gastric upsets; use with chamomile for stress headaches.

If taken regularly it can assist poor circulation; it is actually a useful addition to any herbal medicine for conditions associated with cold and poor circulation. Rosemary treats poor digestion, gall-bladder inflammation, gall stones and liverish feelings.

Preparations

Use it as a gargle for sore throats; it is a useful substitute for sage during pregnancy. Use with horsetail for hair loss due to stress and worry. Two cups of rosemary tea a day will prevent hair loss through poor circulation and re-stimulate growth after chemotherapy. Use the infused oil for massage for cold limbs and aches and pains. Rosemary tea can be used as a conditioning hair rinse for dandruff and for gloriously glossy hair (especially for dark hair) use rosemary vinegar.

Nettle *(Urtica dioica)*

The common stinging nettle – found in the British countryside and many gardens – is often considered a nuisance, but when infused or cooked in soup, it is a useful herbal remedy. It is an iron tonic, mild diuretic and antihistamine.

Strength and Nourishment

Strengthening and styptic, it is useful for iron-deficiency anaemia; nourishing and building, it is good to take in pregnancy or for lethargy, weakness and feelings of heaviness in the body.

It is also good for nettle rash, allergies to strawberries and insect bites; use it also as a tea and a lotion. Nettle can relieve urinary gravel and water retention and be helpful in arthritis. Leave to infuse for 15 minutes for the best effect. The tops can be cooked as spinach or made into soup.

Aloe Vera

Known as Kumari in Ayurvedic medicine, Aloe Vera is used in many therapeutic disciplines, including Western herbalism, folk medicine and Ayurveda. The gel and the leaves of the Aloe Vera plant are used therapeutically.

Aloe Gel

The gel is normally used for healing, while the latex of the leaves is a powerful cleansing agent and a laxative. In Ayurveda, Aloe Vera is used for all three doshas to bring balance. It can relieve inflammation, soothe muscle spasms, purify the blood and cleanse the liver. Fresh Aloe gel, scooped or extracted from the spongy leaves of the plant, can be spread on the skin to heal burns, scalds, scrapes, sunburn and wounds. Apply the gel directly to the outer eyelid to treat conjunctivitis.

Drink the Aloe juice for internal conditions, apply the gel externally. To soothe wounds, clean first with soap and water. Cut several inches off an older leaf, slice it lengthways and apply the gel to the wound. Allow it to dry. You can then leave the gel on the wound for several hours, or wash it off and reapply if it is painful.

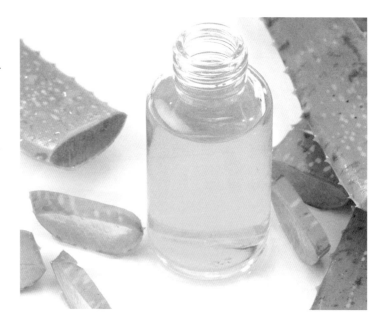

Words of Warning

Aloe gel can cause skin irritation in some people. If irritation persists, discontinue use. Aloe Vera contains a powerful laxative, anthraquinone, which can cause diarrhoea and intestinal cramps. If you use Aloe juice or supplements as a laxative, do it under the guidance of a physician and never exceed the recommended dosage. Commercially packaged products use stabilized Aloe which has none of the fresh herb's healing properties.

Angelica
(*Angelica archangelica* and *A. sinensis*)

In the West, Angelica has been associated with magic and sorcery for centuries. Necklaces of Angelica leaf were thought to provide protection against spells and illness, and its presence in a garden or cupboard was a defence against charges of witchcraft. Fresh Angelica roots are poisonous so they must be dried to eliminate all hazard. Do not use with hypertension or heart disease. Pregnant women should avoid the overuse of Angelica.

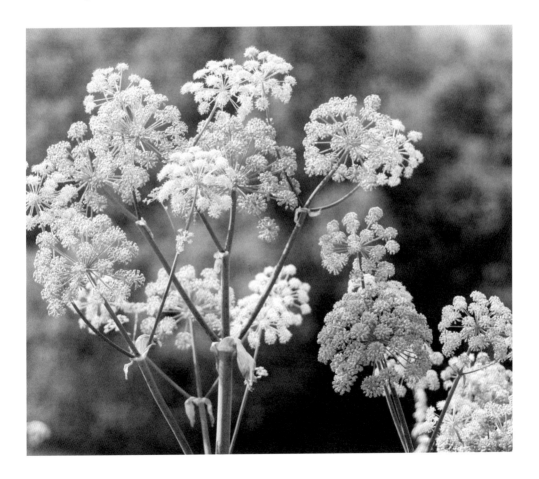

Ayurvedic Angelica

Ayurvedic practitioners prescribe the herb for menstrual problems, as well as arthritis, abdominal pains and flu. In Ayurveda, Angelica balances all three doshas. It is a wonderful expectorant and digestive aid. Prepare the leaves and seeds as an infusion for a mild treatment, or use the root in a decoction for a stronger effect.

Western Angelica

Western herbalists use Angelica for convalescence, persistent fevers, indigestion and weak digestion in general, colic and cramping pains, coughs, poor circulation and general weakness with feelings of cold. Angelica is pungent and sweet, heating and moisturizing. It is a stimulant, expectorant, tonic, emmenagogue, carminative and diaphoretic. Angelica has antibacterial properties, and has been used to induce menstruation and abortion.

Infusions and Decoctions

For an infusion, use one teaspoon of the powdered leaves or seeds in a cup or teapot. Add one cup of boiling water. Steep for 10–15 minutes, then strain. For a decoction, take three teaspoons of the powdered root. Add three cups of water and bring to the boil. Cover and simmer for five minutes. Remove from the heat and let stand for 15 minutes.

Skullcap
(*Scutellaria lateriflora* or *S. galericulata*)

This is one of the main sedative herbs, but it also has a tonic effect on the entire nervous system. It strengthens and calms the nervous system and is antispasmodic. It relieves anxiety, tension headaches, PMS, examination nerves and post-examination depression.

Use with valerian or chamomile and linden flowers for insomnia, disturbed sleep and for tranquillizer withdrawal. Use with vervain for workaholics; the mixture is relaxing without sedating. Skullcap is used as a supportive treatment in epilepsy and for people on major tranquillizers; it reduces anxiety without interfering with medication.

Eyebright *(Euphrasia officinalis)*

Herbalists use the leaves and stems of eyebright (also known by its botanical name *Euphrasia*) either internally or externally. It can work as a tea to help strengthen eye muscles and can also help with problems associated with the upper respiratory tract. Euphrasia can be used as an eye wash to prevent secretion of fluids and relieve discomfort from eye-strain or minor irritation. It is also good for allergies, itchy and/or watery eyes, and runny nose and can help combat hay fever. It is good for congested catarrhal conditions and as an antiseptic for glue ear and sinusitis.

Preparing Euphrasia

Use 1 ml of tincture diluted in water, or one teaspoon of the herb infused in a cup of boiling water. For external use, add two to three drops of tincture in an egg cup of freshly boiled, cooled water.

Gotu Kola *(Centella asiatica)*

The natives of Sri Lanka were the first to use gotu kola. In Ayurvedic medicine, it was used for many skin diseases, including leprosy. Today it is used to aid a variety of conditions: it aids in the elimination of excess fluids, decreases fatigue and depression; it increases sex drive, shrinks tissues and stimulates the central nervous system. It may neutralize blood acids and lower body temperature.

Internal Effects

Gotu kola aids heart and liver function and is useful for cardiovascular and circulatory disorders, fatigue, connective tissue disorders, kidney stones, poor appetite and sleep disorders.

Words of Warning

Some individuals may experience minor irritation or a skin rash when taking gotu kola. Others have experienced headaches. Should such side-effects occur, lessen or discontinue use.

Seeds

Although other parts of these plants and herbs are also used in herbal remedies, the seeds are among the most therapeutic elements, often having a warming and expectorant effect, calming inflammation and easing pain.

Fennel *(Foeniculum vulgare)*

The berries, roots and stems of this familiar cooking herb are used in therapeutic treatment. Warming, carminative, antispasmodic, antidepressant, it promotes milk flow in nursing mothers. It can ease colic, wind and irritable bowel syndrome (IBS), alleviate anxiety, depression and disturbed spirits. Fennel is also known to relieve arthritis and water retention. It can aid griping in infants.

Dosage

For babies, give the tea in teaspoon doses, as much as they will take, or add two teaspoons to milk formulas. Fennel-seed tea bags are easily available. Use one teaspoon of crushed seed to a cup of boiling water and infuse for 10 minutes. Take three times daily.

Mustard *(Sinapis alba, Brassica nigra)*

Mustard is an annual plant cultivated as a spice all over the world. It has been used for centuries as a pungent condiment and healing herb by the Chinese, the Greeks and the Ayurvedics. Black and white mustards are used for culinary and medicinal purposes.

Rubifacient Properties

The leaves, flowers, seeds and oils of the black mustard are used, while only the seeds of the white mustard are useful. Black mustard powder is an important herbal remedy because it draws blood to the surface of the skin quickly, making it rubefacient and warming. Its rubefacient qualities make it useful for respiratory and circulatory disorders.

Aniseed *(Pimpinella anisum)*

Aniseed works mainly on the stomach, intestines and lungs, and its powerful oil is extracted for a wide variety of therapeutic uses.

Expectorant, antispasmodic, carminative, antimicrobial and aromatic, the volatile oil in aniseed provides the basis for its internal use to ease griping, intestinal colic and flatulence. It also has an expectorant and antispasmodic action and may be used for bronchitis, for tracheitis where there is persistent irritable coughing, and for whooping cough. Externally, the oil may be used in an ointment base for the treatment of scabies; the oil by itself will help in the control of lice.

Milk Thistle *(Silybum marianum)*

The mature seeds of the head of the milk thistle plant are used therapeutically. Its properties include:

 Hepatic

 Galactogogue (encourages milk production)

 Demulcent (forms soothing film over mucous membrane)

 Cholagogue (promotes bile flow)

Lactation, Liver and Gall Bladder

Milk thistle is primarily used to promote milk secretion, but it is also exceptionally good for the liver, making it work more efficiently by stabilizing liver-cell membranes and preventing damage from toxins. Milk thistle can be used to increase the secretion and flow of bile from the liver and gall bladder – its traditional use as a liver tonic has been supported by research showing that it contains constituents that protect liver cells from chemical damage; it is used in a whole range of liver and gall-bladder conditions, including hepatitis and cirrhosis. It may also have value in the treatment of chronic uterine problems.

Roots and Bulbs

The roots and bulbs of plants have been used in traditional medicine for centuries – from ubiquitous garlic to exotic kava kava. The beneficial effects of roots such as ginger and bulbs such as garlic are still harnessed all over the world.

Ginger

Ginger is native to India, where the ancient Ayurvedics used it to preserve food, as a digestive aid, and as a spiritual and physical cleanser.

Qualities of Ginger

Ginger is a pungent, sweet herb with warming and drying qualities. It acts as a stimulant, a diaphoretic, an antidepressant and expectorant; ginger stimulates all tissues of the body and is highly recommended in cases where the illness is due to poor assimilation.

Ginger is a muscle relaxant and soothes menstrual cramps. It relieves nausea, particularly during pregnancy, and travel sickness. It is also good for wind, colic and irritable bowel syndrome (IBS). It can be used to treat chills, colds and poor circulation; for fevers, add it to elderflower or yarrow tea. Ginger can be added to most remedies to improve absorption and activity.

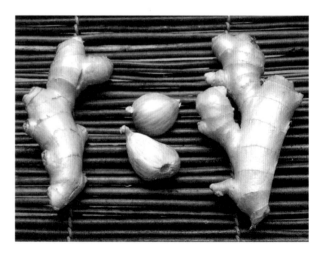

Garlic *(Allium sativum)*

Garlic belongs to the onion family, and is one of the best-known and most-used medicinal herbs. It has a strong odour, which many people find off-putting, but its health-giving and preventative properties make it well worth suffering the effects.

Internal Effects

Garlic is antioxidant and decongestant. It cleanses the blood and helps to create and maintain healthy bacteria (flora) in the gut, as well as treating infections of the stomach and respiratory system. It can help to bring down a fever, reduce high blood pressure and may prevent some cancers. It is known to help prevent heart disease and reduce the risk of atherosclerosis, by toning the heart and circulatory system. Garlic boosts the immune system and may reduce attacks of allergic asthma and hay fever. It is also an antiseptic with antibiotic and antifungal actions.

Garlic Preparations

Fresh garlic, eaten daily, can reduce chronic acidity of the stomach and will reduce the need for antibiotics. Infused oil can be used as a chest rub for respiratory or digestive ailments. Garlic syrup can be used to treat bronchitis, lung infections and digestive disorders. The intestinal tract can be cleansed by adding several mashed, raw garlic cloves to salads.

Dandelion *(Taraxacum officinale)*

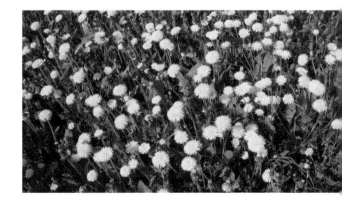

The leaves, flowers and the roots of the common dandelion are a mainstay of herbal medicine, and are best known for their tonic and diuretic properties. The fresh leaves are very nourishing.

Dandelion is an excellent diuretic and kidney tonic and it cleanses by neutralizing the acids in the blood. Dandelion-root coffee is an excellent liver tonic, and can be used in chronic and acute liver conditions; it can also be decocted and used to treat and prevent gallstones. The fresh white sap of the stalks will eliminate warts when used regularly.

Burdock *(Arctium lappa* or *A. minus)*

Burdock is a common wayside plant with large leaves and purple flowers. Both the root and the leaves are used, and both are antimicrobial. It is most commonly used for skin diseases, such as acne, or dry, scaly skin conditions. It acts by pushing toxins out on to the surface of the skin, but it can be given as a diuretic to help flush out toxins from the liver and kidneys.

Uses of Burdock

Burdock is good for rheumatism and gout; it also lowers blood-sugar levels, making it very useful for diabetes. Many people use it to treat eruptive and stubborn skin conditions, especially when hot and inflamed: acne, spots, boils and rashes, psoriasis. Used with dandelion root it can be effective in treating skin and liver problems.

How to Take Burdock

For chronic cystitis and loss of appetite take two teaspoons of dried root, decocted, daily or one teaspoon of the tincture twice daily for some months. For lack of appetite take the tincture three times daily, before meals, in a little water or fruit juice: 5–10 drops for children and 20 drops for adults.

Liquorice *(Glycyrrhiza glabra)*

Native to the Mediterranean region and parts of Asia, liquorice, a pretty blue flower, is cultivated worldwide. The sweet substance is obtained mainly from the roots and is used medicinally and as a flavouring. It is cultivated chiefly in the Middle East.

Uses of Liquorice

Liquorice is expectorant, demulcent, anti-inflammatory, antispasmodic and a mild laxative. It can be effective in the treatment of chronic hepatitis and cirrhosis and is good for detoxifying the whole body.

Liquorice is used in allopathic medicine (traditional, non-homeopathic medecine) as a treatment for peptic ulceration; a similar use to its herbal use in gastritis and ulcers, and it can be used in the relief of abdominal colic. It raises blood pressure and can be used in the treatment of low blood pressure. It stimulates the kidneys and bowels.

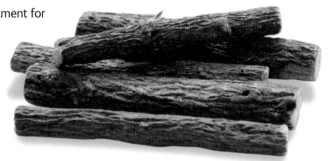

Yellow Dock *(Rumex crispus)*

This nutritious herb helps with poor liver functioning and helps to increase bile flow. It also acts as a laxative for chronic constipation and can be used externally for ringworm or scabies. It treats liver congestion with poor fat digestion and feelings of heaviness after eating. It is also used for stomach acidity and irritable bowel syndrome with constipation.

Use yellow dock for food poisoning and intestinal infections, to clear the source of irritation from the digestive system. Use with burdock for chronic, hot and itchy skin diseases.

Decocting Yellow Dock

Make the decoction using 12 g for 500 ml of water (half an ounce to one pint of water). For constipation one cup of decoction or two teaspoons of tincture daily. More might be needed for short periods. Use half this dose for chronic conditions, for children and for constipation in pregnancy.

Black Cohosh *(Cimicifuga racemosa)*

Also known as black snakeroot, black cohosh is very active in the treatment of rheumatic pains, but also in rheumatoid arthritis, osteoarthritis, in muscular and neurological pain. Black cohosh is also useful in cases of sciatica and neuralgia. As a relaxing nervine it may be used for nervous disorders and stress, and has been found beneficial in cases of tinnitus.

Female Benefits

Black cohosh is a valuable herb with a powerful action as a relaxant and a normalizer of the female reproductive system. It tones the womb and reproductive organs, and brings on menstruation or triggers labour. As it contains oestrogenic substances, this herb is useful for conditions where there is an oestrogen deficiency, such as menopause.

It is an emmenagogue with antispasmodic, alterative, nervine and hypotensive properties. It may be used beneficially in cases of painful or delayed menstruation; ovarian cramps or cramping pain in the womb will be relieved. It helps with the symptoms of PMS, including bloating, pain and emotional symptoms. Black cohosh can give strength to weakened contractions during labour and will help the womb to shrink after childbirth.

Astragalus *(Astragalus membranaceus)*

Used in both Chinese and Western herbalism, astragalus is an important herb for immune function, and for adrenal gland function and digestion.

Huange Qi

In Chinese medicine astragalus is known as Huange Qi and, in that discipline, is widely used for spleen disorders. According to Chinese medicine, astragalus tonifies the spleen and benefits the chi. It also helps water balance problems, such as retention, by regulating the opening and closing of pores and reducing swelling. It is a great tonifier and particularly useful if severe blood loss occurs. It is useful for spleen-deficient symptoms, such as lack of appetite, fatigue and diarrhoea. Its action is upwards and outwards, so it can help with a prolapsed uterus or with uterine bleeding. It is used in prescriptions to help the immune system fight viruses, fight frequent colds and help excessive sweating.

Other Applications

Good for oedema and sores full of pus that have not yet discharged, it is also used in post-partum fever from a severe loss of blood. A decoction or tincture can be used for chronic fatigue, persistent infections, night sweats, multiple allergies and glandular fever. Modern research shows that the herb helps to counteract tiredness and lack of appetite in patients undergoing chemotherapy and radiotherapy for cancer. It is also soothing and healing for stomach ulcers.

Goldenseal *(Hydrastis canadensis)*

This is a powerful antimicrobial and antiseptic herb that has been used in traditional herbal medicine for centuries. Goldenseal acts as an antibiotic, cleanses the body and has anti-inflammatory and antibacterial properties. It increases the effectiveness of insulin and strengthens the immune system; it cleanses mucous membranes, counters infection, improves digestion and regulates periods.

The herb is good for piles and varicose veins, particularly when they are inflamed and bleeding. It is used for catarrhal or infected conditions of the respiratory tract, such as bronchitis or sinusitis.

Goldenseal is a bitter herb which stimulates the liver and digestive system and can be used for loss of appetite, indigestion and constipation. Used at the first sign of symptoms, it can stop colds, flu and sore throats from developing.

Care with Use

Use goldenseal with caution as it can raise blood pressure and may be harsh on the digestive tract. Blend it with other soothing herbs and avoid using it for prolonged periods or during pregnancy. It is not appropriate for those with diabetes, heart disease or glaucoma. It acts as a uterine tonic by increasing circulation to the uterus; it can be given for heavy periods and is useful during labour.

Valerian
(Valeriana officinalis)

This strong-smelling herb is used to relieve conditions that have been induced by anxiety and nervous tension. It is a sedative, nerve restorative, antispasmodic and carminative. Valerian is good for anxiety, confusion, migraines, insomnia and depression with anxiety, useful when flying. It helps palpitations and withdrawal from tranquillizers and is useful in treating high blood pressure due to stress.

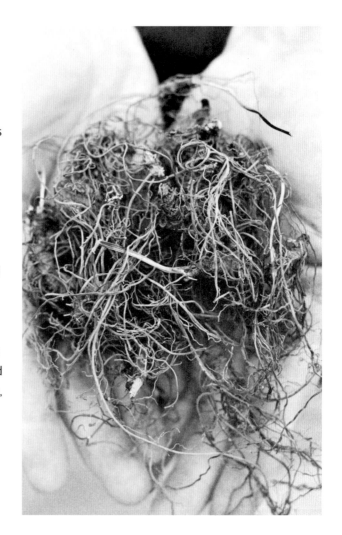

Using Valerian

Use with chamomile for colic and nervous indigestion. The cold decoction is best: soak one teaspoon in a cup of cold water overnight, dose half to one cup. For the tincture, take 20–60 drops three times daily. More may be needed to help tranquillizer withdrawal.

Dong Quai *(Angelica sinensis)*

Chinese angelica, or dong quai, has been used in Asia for thousands of years, and is enjoying renewed popularity as a gynaecological aid. Ayurvedic practitioners prescribe the herb for menstrual problems, as well as arthritis, abdominal pains, and flu. It increases the effects of ovarian and testicular hormones and is used in the treatment of female problems, such as hot flushes and other menopausal symptoms, pre-menstrual syndrome and vaginal dryness.

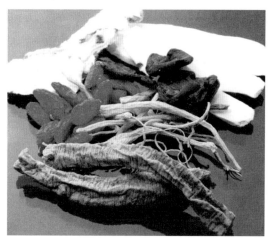

Wild Yam *(Dioscorea villosa)*

Wild yam is the starting point for synthesization of hormones for the contraceptive pill and for 'natural progesterone', which is used in a prescription cream for the menopause. It is anti-inflammatory, antispasmodic and can be used for stomach cramps, nausea, vomiting, hiccups, recurrent colicky pains, pain of diverticulitis and gall bladder pains; use with a little ginger for a quicker action. It is also used for menopausal symptoms and vaginal dryness, and for rheumatoid arthritis. It works especially well on persistent and recurrent problems.

Kava Kava *(Piper methysticum)*

The roots of this powerful herb are used in herbal medicine to induce physical and mental relaxation. It acts as a diuretic and genitourinary antiseptic, and is helpful for anxiety, depression, insomnia, stress-related disorders and urinary tract infections. However, it would be advisable to avoid its use: due to evidence of its link to rare cases of severe liver damage, the Food Standards Agency introduced regulations to ban the sale or distribution of kava kava in England in 2003, and upheld the ban in 2005. Other European countries have done the same.

Bark

The beneficial properties of bark have been a staple of Chinese herbalism and have more recently found their way into the treatments of Western practitioners. It often has warming and comforting properties and can be used for ailments including respiratory problems and cuts and grazes.

Cinnamon *(Cinnamomum zeylanicum)*

Ancient Ayurvedic practitioners used cinnamon as a treatment for fevers, diarrhoea, and as a flavouring for other less-palatable healing herbs. The Greeks used cinnamon to treat bronchitis. Cinnamon is also used in Chinese medicine, but it is not the same plant. Chinese cinnamon, or cassia, is much more powerful and has different uses.

Cinnamon for Healing

Cinnamon is both antiseptic and warming. It is a pungent, sweet astringent, with stimulating, heating qualities; it acts as a diaphoretic, parasiticide, antispasmodic, aphrodisiac, analgesic and diuretic. Cinnamon's antiseptic, antibacterial and antifungal qualities have been frequently utilized in toothpastes and as a treatment for gum disease. As an anti-yeast agent, cinnamon has been used to treat candida and other yeast infections.

Anaesthetic and Antiseptic

Cinnamon contains the natural anaesthetic oil eugenol, which will help relieve the pain of minor wounds. To treat cuts and scrapes, wash the affected area thoroughly and pat dry. Sprinkle powdered cinnamon lightly over the area, then bind or bandage. Repeat treatment as needed until the area is healed. It is also recommended for respiratory ailments such as colds, sinus congestion and bronchitis. As a digestive aid, it relieves dyspepsia, intestinal infections and parasites.

Slippery Elm *(Ulmus fulva)*

The bark of this small American tree is used therapeutically, mainly for its soothing and mucilaginous qualities. It forms a lining over the wall of the stomach, soothing ulcers that are irritated by stomach acid, as in the case of colitis and other inflammatory conditions. Slippery elm is good for any sort of inflammation or irritation in the digestive tract:

 Nausea
 Indigestion
 Wind
 Food allergies
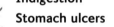 Stomach ulcers
 Acidity
 Heartburn
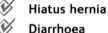 Hiatus hernia
Colitis
Diverticulitis
Diarrhoea

Usage

Mix with sufficient water to make a paste for drawing splinters. Tablets flavoured with carminative herbs are especially useful. Take one or two with a glass of water or milk before meals. For travel sickness and nausea during pregnancy suck one tablet slowly.

Comfrey *(Symphytum officinale)*

Comfrey is a common wild plant with large bristly leaves and clusters of purple flowers; the root is used for treatment. Comfrey promotes rapid healing of cuts, wounds, sprains and broken bones. It can be taken as a tea or tincture and used in poultices, creams and liniments. It is particularly useful with chamomile and meadowsweet for hiatus hernia and stomach ulcers.

Comfrey ointment is a traditional soothing and healing preparation for sprains and aches and pains. Add a few drops of a warming essential oil, such as black pepper, to the infused oil to make a good liniment for arthritis, bunions and aches and pains arising from old injuries.

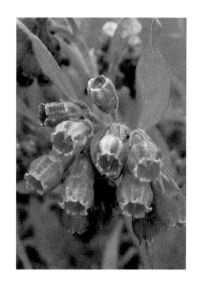

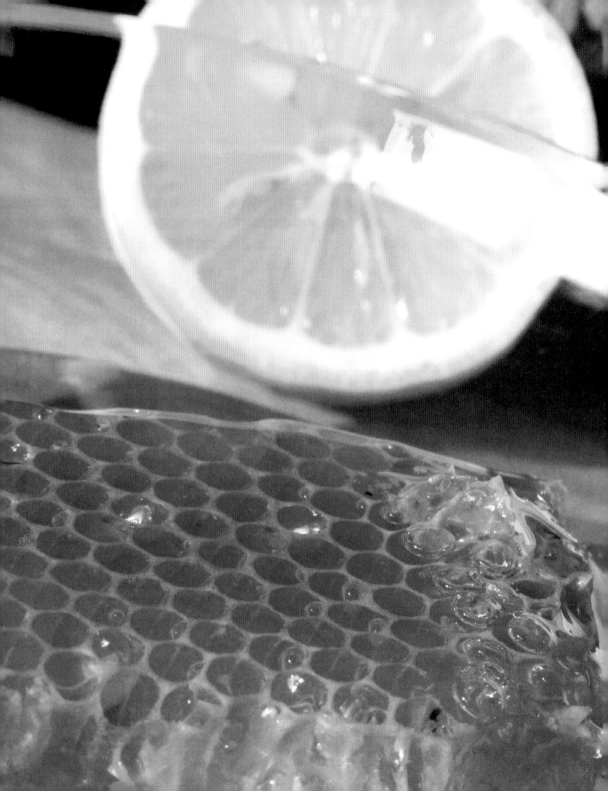

home remedies

History of Home Remedies

Since the beginning of civilization, people have turned to nature to find ways of healing the body, mind and soul. Healers in various tribes and communities were once greatly revered for their methods and medicines, and these people used only the natural remedies available to them to provide effective ways of healing.

Ancient Practices

Many ancient societies produced highly evolved systems of medicine, as can be seen from the Ayurvedic practices in India and traditional Chinese medicine in China, both of which were based on natural remedies and holistic methods of diagnosis and treatment. In many parts of the world, these practices continue today, and it is estimated that 80 per cent of the world's population still rely on plants as their first form of medicine.

The Decline of Natural Healing

Until the beginning of the twentieth century, almost every family used items already in the home to treat minor ailments and medical emergencies, from the common cold to cuts and grazes – honey to soothe sore throats or bread to make poultices, for example. Recipes for family medicines and cures were passed down the generations.

With the advent of modern medicine, however, these practices declined. More people had access to doctors and formal medical advice. Pills were available that seemed to cure all manner of ailments, although in reality these medicines treated the symptoms rather than the cause of the illness. People stopped using natural products and instead relied on manufactured treatments dispensed by medical professionals. They began to lose touch with their bodies, relying on others to treat them.

Resurgence of Home Remedies

As the flaws in the conventional medical system became more obvious, however, there has been a renewed interest in natural healing, and in particular, home remedies. The fact is that there are many ailments that can be treated at home with many herbs, plants and fruits that are often already in the cupboard. From lemons and grapefruits, through onions, cabbage and carrots to all sorts of herbs and spices, much natural produce has great healing qualities which, when applied correctly in the right amounts, can prove extremely effective.

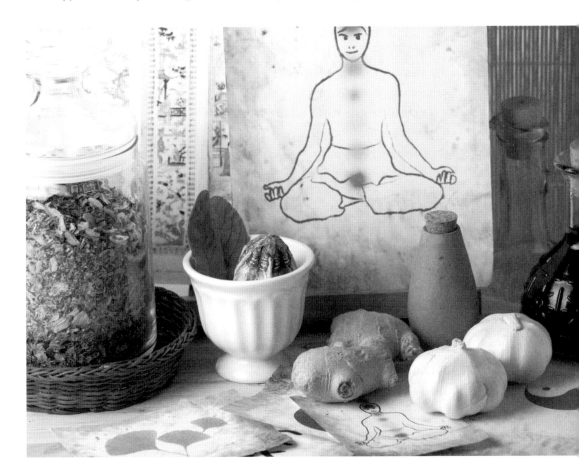

Fruit

The value of citrus fruit – packed with vitamin C – to fight off colds has long been known and used. However, fruit is full of other powerful healing agents and can act as a detoxifier, antiseptic and can even be used in poultices to draw out infections.

Apple *(Malus species)*

Apple has many uses in traditional medicine and the old adage 'to eat an apple going to bed, will make the doctor beg his bread' has been justified by its many health-giving properties. Modern research shows that apples are excellent detoxifiers and apple juice – even from the supermarket shelf – can destroy viruses in the body. Pay attention, however, to how many apple seeds you actually ingest, as they can be toxic when taken in large amounts.

Uses for Apple

Apple cleans the teeth and strengthens gums, lowers cholesterol levels, protects from pollution by binding to toxins in the body and carrying them out, neutralizes indigestion and prevents constipation. Apples also have an antiviral action and are soothing, with antiseptic properties.

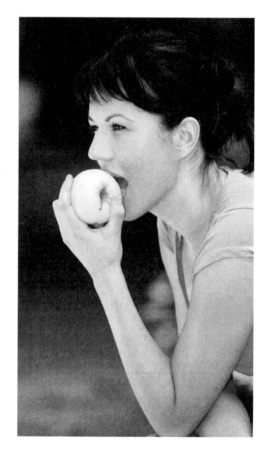

How to Use

To prevent viruses from settling in and to reduce their duration, eat an apple (or a glass of apple juice) three times a day. Raw, peeled and grated apples can be used as a poultice for sprains. For indigestion, heartburn and other digestive disorders, eat an apple with meals. Use as a poultice for rheumatic and weak eyes. Two apples a day can reduce cholesterol levels by up to 10 per cent. As a treatment for intestinal infections, hoarseness, rheumatism and fatigue, increase your daily intake to up to 1 kg. For curative purposes, as an alternative to eating the whole fruit, drink 600 ml of naturally sweet apple juice a day. Grated apple, mixed with live yoghurt, may be helpful in cases of diarrhoea.

Lemon *(Citrus limon)*

Lemons are the most widely grown acid species belonging to the citrus group of fruits. They rank third in tonnage among all citrus fruit produced and have, for generations, been used for their wide range of therapeutic properties and uses. Lemons are a rich source of vitamins C and B, and have a cleansing effect on the digestive system. They are the mainstay of any good 'home remedy' chest. The leaves and the whole fruit may be used according to requirements.

Properties of Lemon

Lemon is a blood purifier, it improves the body's ability to expel toxins and is useful for skin problems such as acne and boils. Lemon is antifungal, antacid, antiseptic and a good digestive aid, they are thus excellent for halting the progress of infections. The high potassium content of lemons will encourage the heart action and lemons are a useful tonic for anyone with heart problems.

Benefits of Lemon Juice

Drink fresh lemon juice (lemon in hot water will do) to cleanse the system. Lemon strengthens the immune system, helps relieve the symptoms of colds and flu and can also be beneficial in the treatment of other infections. Use pure lemon juice on wasp stings to relieve pain. Regular intake of fresh lemons may be useful in the treatment of haemorrhoids, kidney stones and varicose veins. Lemon juice mixed with olive oil may help to dissolve gallstones. To help cure cold sores put a few drops of undiluted lemon juice on the affected area and repeat several times a day until the sore disappears.

Grapefruit *(Citrus paradisi)*

Like all citrus fruit, grapefruit is rich in vitamin C and potassium. Pink grapefruit is rich in vitamin A, and acts as a natural antioxidant. Grapefruit is an excellent cleanser for the digestive and urinary systems. It aids the break-up of fats in the body, strengthens the respiratory system and aids respiration. It is also known to relieve symptoms of cold and flu, balance the nervous system and may help in the treatment of osteoarthritis.

Peel and Pips

The peel has many therapeutic properties. Grapefruit pith and membranes lower cholesterol in the blood and grapefruit seeds can be eaten to rid the body of worms.

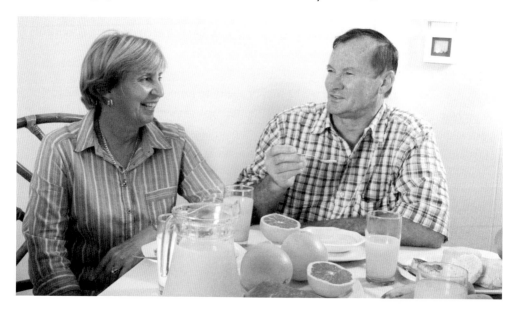

Juice

Drinking grapefruit juice can encourage healthy skin – used in the treatment of acne for its mild exfoliating properties. The juice cleanses the kidneys and rids the body of toxins. Drinking grapefruit juice with iron supplements, or foods rich in iron, increases the absorption of iron in the body. It detoxifies the liver, can ease chronic liver conditions and may help to reduce the severity of a hangover.

Essential Oil

Grapefruit essential oil is popular in aromatherapy. Local massage with a few drops of essential oil in a carrier oil will relieve headaches; it is also invigorating and uplifting, and may help to treat depression. A massage stimulates the immune system, which is particularly useful when suffering from infections.

Rhubarb
(Rheum palmatum and R. officinale)

There are several different types of rhubarb. Chinese rhubarb is also known as 'turkey rhubarb'. Garden rhubarb is a hybrid. Rhubarb has several properties and uses:

- **Laxative**
- **Astringent**
- **Bitter tonic**
- **Cooling**
- **Alleviates constipation, acute liver and gall-bladder diseases, feelings of congestion and fullness in the stomach**
- **Treats stomach acidity, gastroenteritis and diarrhoea from food poisoning and gout**
- **Used in cancer treatments**
- **Uses as a poultice for abscesses**

Rhubarb Decoction

To make a decoction use half a teaspoon to a cup of water or, for the tincture, use 30–40 drops, three times daily.

Cranberry *(Vaccinium oxycoccos var. palustris)*

Cranberries are small acidic berries that are rich in vitamin C and contain an excellent infection-fighting ingredient. They also contain large amounts of oxalic acid and should not be eaten raw. Cranberries improve the health of the circulatory system. They contain a substance that affects the acidity of the urine and acts as a bactericide; a daily glass of cranberry juice will prevent and treat cystitis and discourage kidney stones. Crushed cranberries, boiled in distilled water and skinned, can be added to a cup of warm water to overcome an asthma attack; the berries contain an active ingredient similar to the drugs used to control asthma.

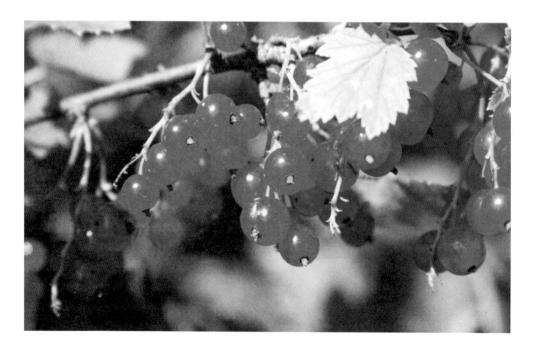

Avocado *(Persea americana gratissima)*

Avocados are the fruit of a small, sub-tropical tree. They are rich in vitamins A, some B-complex, C and E, potassium and antioxidants. Because they contain some protein and starch, as well as being a good source of monounsaturated fats, avocados are considered to be a perfect, or complete, food. Do not eat avocados or take any product containing avocado if you have been prescribed the antidepressants monoamine oxidase inhibitors (MAOI).

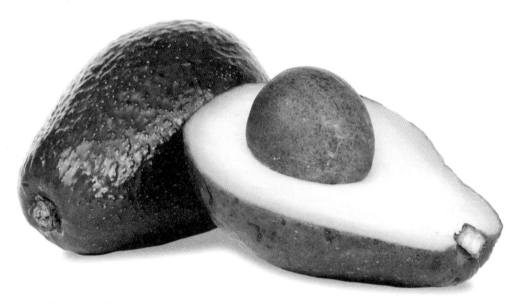

Home Uses for Avocado

Traditionally avocados have been used for skin problems. The pulp has both antibacterial and antifungal properties and can prevent infection when applied to grazes and shallow cuts. It is a restorative food, particularly during convalescence. It has traditionally been used for sexual problems, skin disorders and to treat circulatory problems. It also aids the digestive system.

Avocado oil can be used as a base oil for massage. Eat avocado regularly to help alleviate symptoms of digestive and circulatory problems. The flesh of a ripe avocado soothes sunburnt skin; cut in half and rub gently over the affected area.

Vegetables

There are many applications for vegetables in treating minor ailments. They can help fight off colds, reduce cholesterol, or made into poultices to draw out infections. This is in addition to the health benefits of simply making a variety of vegetables part of your everyday diet.

Onion *(Allium cepa)*

Onions have long been considered the mainstay of every household remedy chest as they are expectorant, antibacterial and diuretic. The bulb of the onion is used in cooking and medicinally.

Warming and Healing

Like garlic, it warms the body and stimulates the circulation; its stimulating effect also aids the secretion of digestive juices. Onion juice has been used to treat infected wounds, amoebic dysentery, and, at one time, juice applied to the ear was said to cure deafness! It can help to reduce serum cholesterol after a fatty meal and, mixed with honey, can relieve the symptoms of a cold. Onions may even provide some protection against cancer.

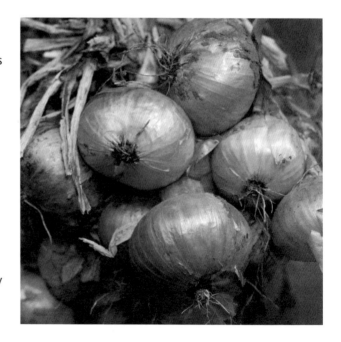

Applying Onions

Onion may be used directly on the skin for natural relief from burns; simply place slices of raw onion on the burnt skin, or apply a homemade lotion of onion juice mixed with salt; this preparation is also effective for insect bites and stings. For an antibiotic treatment, peel and eat (raw or cooked) one quarter of one sweet white onion, two to four times a day; the onion must be chewed, crushed, chopped or bruised to access its antibiotic effects. Onion poultices are used to treat bronchitis and can also help in the treatment of acne and boils. Use a poultice of roasted onion for earache.

Carrot *(Daucus carota)*

A member of the Umbelliferae family, which also includes celery and parsnip, the carrot is a widely grown vegetable. Carrots were first used as medicinal herbs rather than as vegetables, and today they have the dual purpose of acting as therapeutic agents and providing the best source of betacarotene (a form of vitamin A) in the human diet. They are rich in vitamins A, B, C and E and the minerals phosphorus, potassium and calcium.

Cabbage *(Brassica oleracea)*

Cabbage has traditionally been used for medicinal purposes as well as for cooking. It has anti-inflammatory properties and contains chemicals that can prevent cancer.

Ancient Applications

The ancient Greeks used fresh white cabbage juice to relieve sore or infected eyes, and cabbage juice from the stem is a good remedy for ulcers. Traditionally, the Romans and Egyptians would drink cabbage juice before big dinners to prevent intoxication; cabbage seeds are said to prevent hangovers. It has several other uses. Cabbage contains lactic acid, which acts to disinfect the colon, soothe eczema and reduce the pain of headaches and rheumatic disorders.

Home Remedies

Red cabbage leaves form the basis of a good cough syrup. A cabbage poultice can be applied to boils and infected cuts to draw out the infection and disperse pus. Applied to bruises and swelling, macerated cabbage leaves will encourage healing. Dab white cabbage juice on mouth ulcers and gargle for sore throats. A warm cabbage compress on the affected area will reduce headaches and some neuralgias. Drink fresh cabbage juice to reduce the discomfort of gastric ulcers and bronchial infections. A cabbage leaf, lightly pounded, can be placed directly on the breast to relieve mastitis.

Cayenne *(Capsicum annuum)*

This fiery red pepper, used all over the world in cooking, is known to many Westerners by its Caribbean name, cayenne. It is widely used in Ayurvedic medicine, and has warming and mucus-relieving qualities. Use rubber gloves when chopping cayenne peppers, as they may burn the fingertips. If burning should occur, wash with vinegar several times, rinsing carefully.

Properties of Cayenne

Cayenne acts as a decongestant and an expectorant, and alleviates colds, gastrointestinal and bowel problems; it is used as a digestive aid by stimulating the flow of saliva and stomach secretions. It has analgesic and warming properties, increasing circulation; it also has strong digestive, carminative and emetic properties. It can be used as a treatment for colds, fever, toothache, diarrhoea and constipation. Creams containing cayenne are frequently used in the treatment of shingles.

Celery *(Apium graveolens)*

Hippocrates, the father of medicine, wrote that celery could be used to calm the nerves, and indeed, its very high calcium level is likely the reason for this phenomenon. The seeds, leaves and edible root of the plant are used.

Juice and Seeds

Celery is best eaten raw, and its juice is particularly useful. The seeds are rich in iron and many vitamins, including A, B and C, and can be used in the treatment of liver problems, high blood pressure and to ease insomnia. Celery seeds are used by Ayurvedic practitioners to reduce indigestion, a nervous stomach and ungrounded emotions.

In aromatherapy, celery seed oil can be used to counteract jet lag, and exposure to smog and toxic environments. Celery may help in the treatment of arthritis and rheumatic disorders; as it clears uric acid from painful joints. Grated, raw celery can be used as a poultice for swollen glands. Celery root is said to be an aphrodisiac.

Cucumber
(Cucumis sativus)

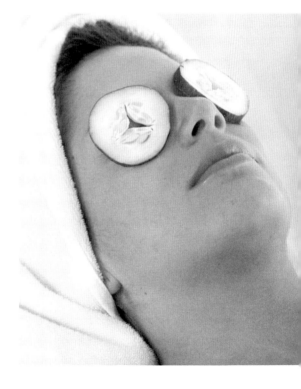

The cucumber is a vine fruit that can be eaten fresh or pickled. Cucumber has been widely used in folk medicine to reduce heat and inflammation. It is a rich source of vitamin C and can be used externally to cool and cleanse, making it particularly good for skin disorders and in the treatment of gout and arthritis. Drink cucumber juice or eat fresh cucumber to soothe heartburn or an acid stomach; drink 100–150 ml every two hours for a gastric or duodenal ulcer. Place a cucumber slice over strained or inflamed eyes to reduce swelling and soothe. Apply fresh cucumber or cucumber juice to sunburn to cool. Ground dried cucumber seeds are used to treat tapeworm. Cucumber juice, drunk daily, may help to control eczema and can act as a kidney tonic.

Grains

Barley and oats are both rich in nutrients, but they can both be used therapeutically. They have a warming and cleansing effect, and can be used to treat a variety of ailments, including depression, nervous exhaustion, constipation and eczema.

Barley *(Hordeum sativum vulgare)*

Barley is rich in minerals (calcium and potassium) and B-complex vitamins, which make it useful for convalescents, or people suffering from stress. Barley has been used for its restorative qualities, in medicine and in cooking, for thousands of years. Malt is produced from barley. It is anti-inflammatory – particularly for the urinary and digestive systems. Taken daily, it may lower cholesterol levels. Make a poultice of barley flour to reduce inflammation of the skin.

Barley Water

Barley water can be used in the treatment of respiratory disorders, and eases dry, tickling coughs. It is also good for urinary tract infections and cystitis, and can ease flatulence and colic. It reduces acidity in the spleen if drunk twice a day for a month.

Cooked Barley

Cooked barley is easily digested and nutritious, and is a traditional remedy for constipation and diarrhoea. Barley may help to prevent heart disease, as it promotes the normal functioning of the heart and stabilizes blood pressure. Eat it in soups and stews when convalescing.

Oats *(Avena sativa)*

Oats are a cereal plant, and are both extremely nutritious and useful therapeutically. Oats are one of the best sources of Inositol, which is important for maintaining blood cholesterol levels.

They are rich in B vitamins and minerals. Eaten daily, they provide a wealth of excellent effects. Oats do not contain gluten and are therefore appropriate for a gluten-free diet – particularly since they are so nourishing.

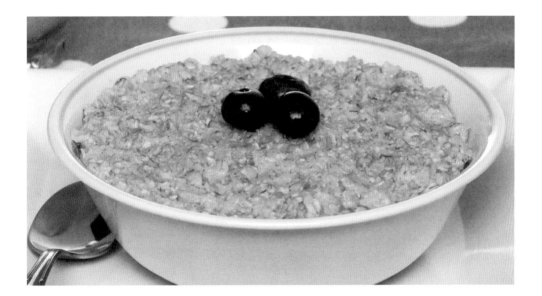

Treatments

Oats can be used as a tonic for general debility, in the treatment of anorexia and for convalescence and fatigue. They can lower blood cholesterol levels and help control hormonal activity. They are cleansing – internally and externally – and may protect against bowel cancer when taken internally. Oats can have an antidepressant effect and can be used to treat depression, stress and nervous disorders; they are often used in the treatment of addictions. Eat raw oats to ease constipation. Oatmeal (unrefined) can be eaten on a regular basis to reduce the effects of stress and nervous disorders; cooked oats will relieve fatigue. A compress of oatmeal, or an oatmeal bath soothes eczema and other skin conditions. Boil a tablespoon of oats in 275 ml or 10 fl oz of water for several minutes and drain; use as a nerve tonic and for its nourishing properties.

From the Larder

Besides fruit and vegetables, a wealth of home remedies can be made from basic ingredients found in the kitchen cupboard or fridge. Oils, vinegars, herbs and spices can all be adapted to treat a variety of ailments.

Bread

Wholegrain bread is an excellent source of carbohydrates and B-complex vitamins, which maintain the health of the nervous system and ensures healthy functioning of body systems. Traditionally, bread was used as a poultice, and applied as a styptic to stop bleeding of wounds. It has many properties: it is nutritious and anti-inflammatory – apply cold bread to closed eyes to reduce the inflammation of conjunctivitis and soothe itching, or a warm bread poultice to infected cuts to reduce itching and pain. Apply fresh bread to shallow wounds to help stop the bleeding. Apply a hot bread poultice to ease the pain of a boil and help bring it out.

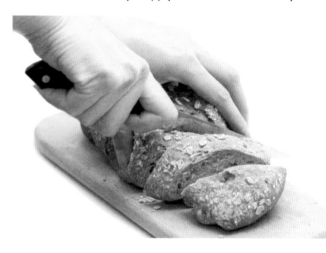

Olive Oil
(Olea europaea)

The leaves of the olive tree are used therapeutically as well as the oil from the fruit. Olive oil is an excellent source of vitamin E; it is high in monounsaturated fats and has a high energy value. Olive oil has a beneficial effect on the circulatory and nervous systems and may reduce the risk of circulatory disease.

Internal and External Effects

Olive oil also benefits the digestive system and those suffering from hyperacidity, as it reduces the level of gastric secretions. The leaves of the olive are used to treat high blood pressure, stress and abrasions. The oil itself can help in the treatment of constipation and peptic ulcers; it is also useful for dry skin and hair, particularly for the treatment of a dry, flaky scalp.

Vinegar *(Acetic acid)*

Vinegar is an acidic liquid obtained from the fermentation of alcohol and used either as a condiment or a preservative. Vinegar usually has an acid content of between four and eight per cent; in flavour it may be sharp, rich or mellow. Vinegar is often used to preserve herbs, and is used on its own for medicinal purposes. Apple cider vinegar is the most useful medicinally.

Properties

Vinegar helps to make more efficient use of calcium in the body, and can help to encourage strong bones, hair and nails. It is antispasmodic, antibacterial, antiseptic, astringent and excellent for urinary tract infections. It improves functioning and adjustment of the body so that there is efficient use of the food you eat. Its anti-fungal properties make it useful in the treatment of thrush.

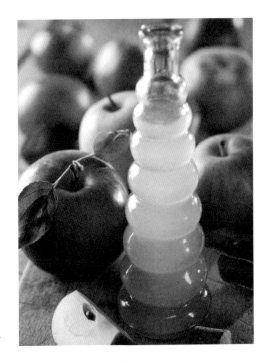

Cider Vinegar

Apple cider vinegar is a good tonic and relieves sore throats. Sip first thing in the morning and just prior to meals to reduce appetite and encourage efficient digestion of food. Simmer cider vinegar in a pan, cover with a towel and inhale to reduce the spasms of bronchitis and to help reduce any excess catarrh. Drink a glass of warm apple cider vinegar with honey half an hour before bed to encourage restful sleep. Vinegar can be drunk (warm, with a little honey) to treat digestive disorders and urinary infections.

Apply vinegar to wasp stings to reduce swelling and ease discomfort. Apply cider vinegar on the skin to treat athlete's foot, ringworm and eczema.

Vinegar Mixtures

Coughs, colds and infections will respond to a cup of warm water with two tablespoons of vinegar and some honey; arthritis and asthma may also be treated with the same drink, adding slightly more vinegar. Drink vinegar daily to treat thrush, and apply to the exterior of the vagina (mixed with a little warm water) to ease itching. Add vinegar to bath water to soothe skin problems, to help draw out toxins from the skin and ease thrush.

Yoghurt

As a food, yoghurt is a rich source of protein and all the vitamins and minerals found in milk. Live yoghurt, which contains active bacteria, is most often used therapeutically and should be eaten to increase the healthy bacteria in the body, which help our body to fight infection. Live yoghurt may help to reduce blood cholesterol levels and should be eaten to increase beneficial bacteria following a course of antibiotics; eat daily for two to three weeks for best effect. Apply live yoghurt to areas affected by thrush; it can also be used internally as a douche. Daily intake of yoghurt may prevent heart disease.

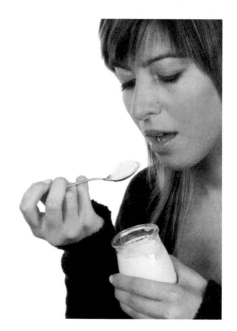

Honey

For centuries honey has been used as an antiseptic, for external and internal conditions, and as a tonic for overall good health. Unpasteurized honey should not be eaten by pregnant women and only sparingly by children. However, ensure that you buy cold-pressed honey because heated honey contains additives and loses its healing effect.

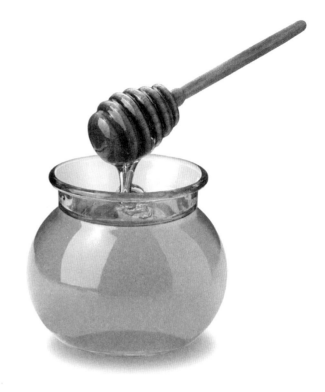

Soothing Properties

Honey soothes raw tissue and helps to retain calcium in the body. It also helps to balance acid accumulations in the body because of the significant amount of potassium it contains. It has anti-sedative and anti-bacterial properties, making it ideal for external and internal infections; there are active antibiotic properties in unpasteurized honey.

Honey water can be used as an eye lotion (particularly good for conjunctivitis and other infective conditions). Gargle with honey water to soothe a sore throat and ease respiratory problems. Honey ointment can soothe and encourage healing of sores in the mouth or vagina. Honey is an excellent moisturiser and can be rubbed into the skin as a revitalizing mask.

Honey Mixtures

Honey and lemon are a traditional remedy for coughs. Mix with apple cider vinegar as a tonic or 'rebalancer'; this concoction may also help to relieve the symptoms of arthritis and reduce arthritic deposits.

Bicarbonate of Soda

Bicarbonate of soda is used in many natural remedies and on its own for its soothing and neutralizing properties. It is anti-inflammatory and particularly useful for skin conditions. A paste of bicarbonate of soda and water can be applied to nappy rash to reduce inflammation and irritation. Drink a solution of bicarbonate of soda and hot water (one teaspoon for every 225 ml) to reduce flatulence and ease indigestion. For bee stings, extract the sting and apply a paste of bicarbonate of soda and water to neutralize. The juice of half a lemon mixed with one teaspoon of bicarbonate of soda and warm water will help ease a headache; drink every 15 minutes until the pain is reduced. Bicarbonate of soda should only be used externally on children and babies.

Turmeric *(Curcuma longa)*

Turmeric holds a place of honour in Ayurvedic medicine. It is a symbol of prosperity, and was believed to be a cleanser for all the systems in the body. Turmeric was prescribed as a digestive aid, a treatment for fever, infections, dysentery, arthritis and jaundice. Its properties are antiseptic, warming and astringent. Do not use in cases of hepatitis or pregnancy. Turmeric is said to reduce fertility, and would not be recommended for someone trying to conceive.

Turmeric Infusions

Turmeric acts as a stimulant, an alterative and carminative with vulnerary (wound-healing) and antibacterial properties. It reduces fat, purifies blood and aids circulation. It can benefit digestion and can help rid the body of intestinal parasites. A turmeric infusion will help all these conditions and reduce arthritic pain. Warm one cup of milk; remove from the heat before boiling; stir in one teaspoon of turmeric powder; drink up to three cups a day.

Cloves *(Eugenia caryophyllata)*

Cloves are antiseptic and analgesic – particularly good for gums and teeth. They are also warming, useful for people who are prone to colds. They have anti-inflammatory properties when used locally on swellings, are calming on the digestive system and can eliminate parasites from the body. They are also a powerful analgesic. Cloves can cause uterine contractions and should not be used in pregnancy.

Clove Oil

Oil of cloves can be chewed or placed directly on a sore tooth or mouth abscess to draw out the infection and ease the pain. A tiny amount of neat oil can be dabbed on insect bites to alleviate the sting. The oil can also be used during a long labour to hasten birth.

Clove Tea

Clove tea is a warming drink and can encourage the body to sweat, which is helpful in cases of high fever. The tea can also be used to soothe wind and ease nausea – particularly travel sickness. The tea is also renowned for helping to lift depression. Inhale an infusion of clove to clear the lungs and refresh. Steep cloves in boiling water, simmer, strain and use the remaining liquid as a mild sedative and to soothe an acid stomach.

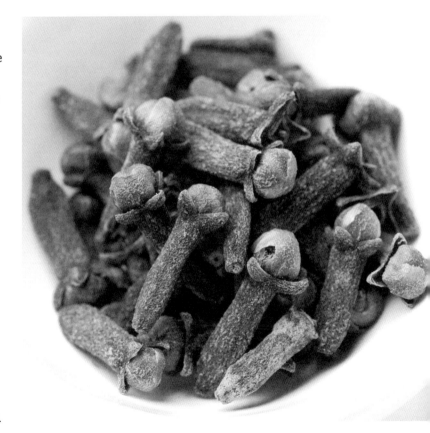

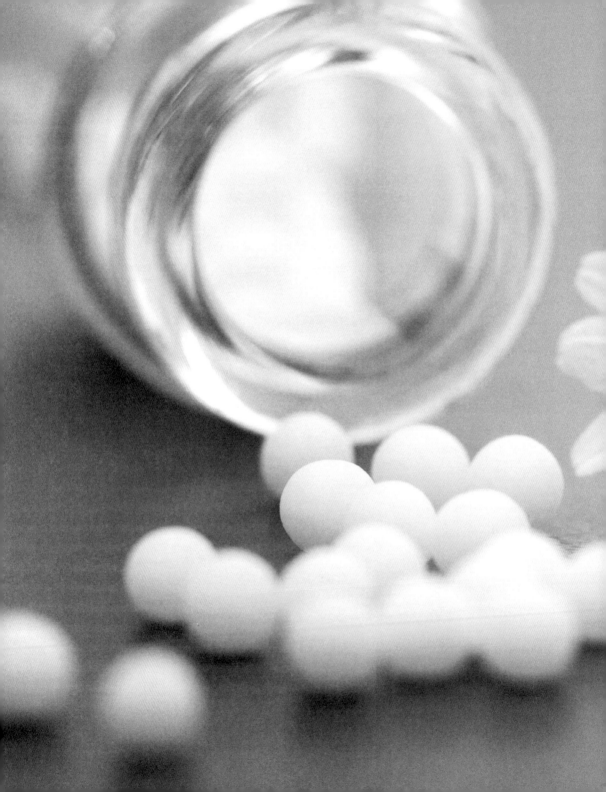

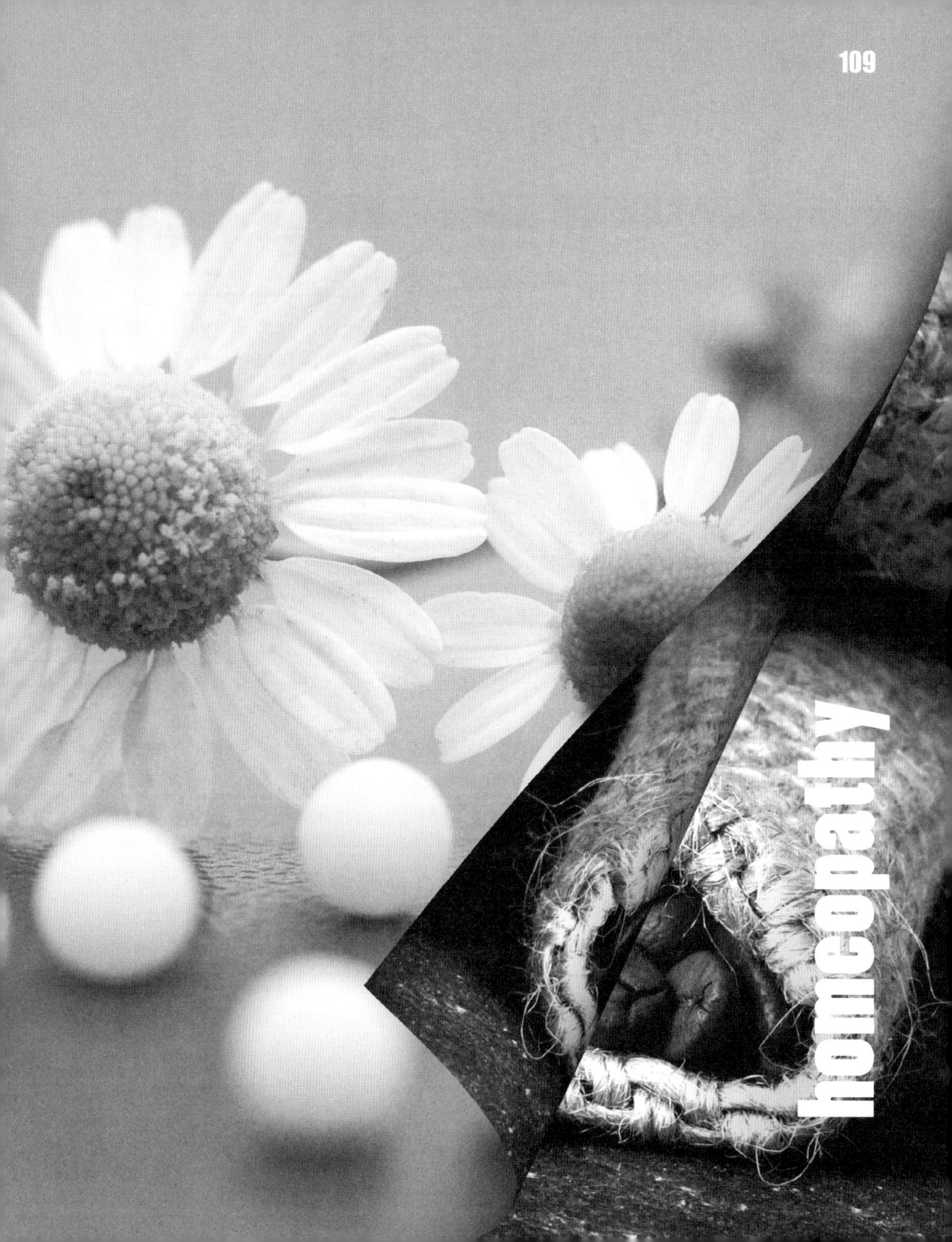

homeopathy

Understanding Homeopathy

Homeopathy is often confused with herbalism, partly, perhaps, because some of the remedies are made with herbs. However, herbalists use material concentrations of plants, while homeopathic remedies use plants, minerals and even some animal products as a base. They are prepared through a process known as potentization to bring out their subtle healing properties.

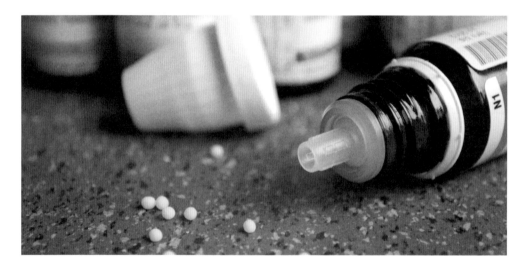

Balancing Energy

We know from modern physics that our seemingly solid bodies are just dense fields of energy. A disturbance in our energy field can give rise to disease, and a potent form of energy can rebalance us. Homeopathy uses potentized remedies to rebalance our body's subtle energy system. Once this is back in balance, the immune system and the other interconnected systems in our body start functioning better.

Symptoms

The term 'homeopathy' comes from the Greek language, meaning 'similar suffering'. It reflects the key principle behind the homeopathic method – that a substance can cure the symptoms in an ill person that it is capable of causing in a healthy person.

Samuel Hahnemann believed that symptoms and signs of an illness are in fact attempts on the part of the body to heal itself, so that when a substance capable of producing a similar symptom 'picture' to that of the disease is used, it encourages a powerful strengthening of the defence mechanism. A homeopath, therefore, must study the entire symptoms picture to get a full idea of the disease and prescribe the correct remedy. Often it is the symptoms that seem almost incidental, strange or rare that are the most valuable to the homeopathic practitioner, for they give the disease its own particular character and thus suggest the remedy.

Safe Use of Homeopathy

You can use homeopathy at home completely safely as long as you follow some simple guidelines.

- **Do not**: Attempt to treat yourself at home if you have serious health problems.

- **Do not**: Use self-help remedies instead of seeing your doctor for a diagnosis, or take yourself off medication without advice.

- **Do not**: Take lots of different remedies at the same time.

- **Do not**: Keep taking homeopathic remedies indefinitely, as this can aggravate your symptoms if the remedy is not appropriate for you.

- **Do not**: Take high potencies (200 and over) of remedies unless prescribed by a registered homeopath. Remember that these potencies work on an emotional as well as physical level and your symptoms may require only physical treatment. You may bring on a whole host of unwanted effects by choosing too high a potency and compound the problem rather than solving it.

Homeopathic Remedies

A homeopathic remedy is an extremely pure, natural substance that has been diluted many times. In large quantities these substances would cause the same symptoms that the patient is trying to cure. In small, diluted doses, it is not only safe and free from side-effects, but it will trigger the body to heal itself.

Many scientists have claimed that a study of the remedies themselves has proved that there is little or even no trace of the original substance in the tablet. This is the basis of the scientific assertion that homeopathy effects cure through positive thinking alone. Do not be fooled by these claims. Homeopathy is an extremely subtle medicine, based on the concept of 'vibrational medicine'. Because the remedies are so diluted, they often contain only a

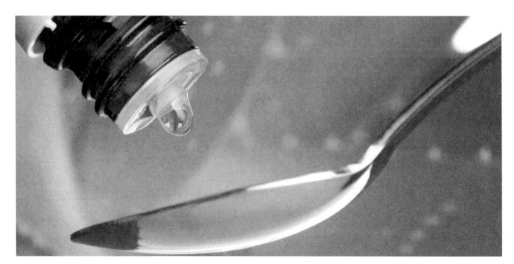

vibration of the original substance, and it is this vibration that works on the body's natural energy field. It is like a radio signal rather than an overt substance, but it is that subtle signal which effects a cure.

Potency Levels

Homeopathic remedies are classified into three levels of potency; X, C and M refer to 10, 100 and 1,000 in terms of the amount of dilution. The more a tincture is diluted, the more potent it becomes. So, while a C is more dilute than an X, the C is more powerful. M-classified remedies are extremely potent and are normally prescribed by homeopathic practitioners on a constitutional basis.

Constitutional Types

Most people, when they are ill, do not only suffer from the basic symptoms of the disease but other symptoms that are specific to them. These additional symptoms are vital for choosing the right remedy. This is why some patients may receive different remedies for the same disease.

Many homeopaths noticed that different types of people reacted strongly to certain remedies and proposed that people should be placed in different categories, known as 'constitutional types'. This is why a homeopath will say that someone is a 'sulphur type' or 'obviously a Calc Carb'. This basically means that people react strongly to these remedies. The belief is that people of one type share similarities in terms of body shape, character, personality, and the type of diseases to which they succumb. For instance, lycopodium types tend to be tall and stooped with an anxious expression and a craving for sweets.

The Big Picture

Constitutional types are useful, but certainly not the only criteria for prescribing treatment. Constitutional treatment means looking at the whole picture of a person's health, from inherited predisposition, past illnesses, diet, general reactions to the environment, intellectual

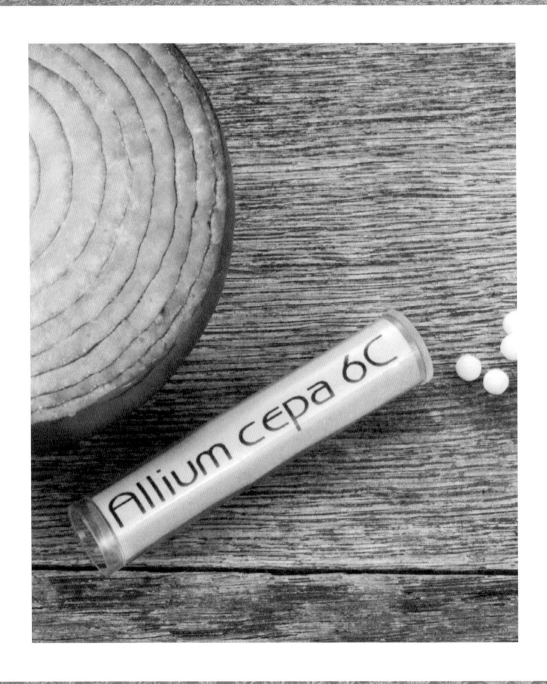

and emotional features, and general attitude to life. This is constitutional treatment, which differs, of course, to labelling someone as a constitutional type.

Key Notes

It is important to understand how homeopathic remedies work and to use them correctly.

- **Forms**: Remedies come in tablet form, or as granules for young children. Tinctures and creams are also available.

- **Potency**: The number printed on the label of any homeopathic medicine you buy indicates how many times it has been diluted and succussed (shaken firmly). A 6 potency has been diluted six times, while a 30 has been diluted 30 times.

- **Dosage**: One tablet (or a few granules) is enough for one dose. Dissolve the tablet under your tongue without water. Crush tablets in paper for small children or babies, and try to avoid touching it with your own hands.

- **Children**: Children can have a tablet dissolved in a small quantity of water, but again, do not touch the remedy with your own hands.

- **After taking**: Do not eat, drink, clean your teeth or smoke for at least 20 minutes before or afterwards, in case any strong substances in your mouth spoil the effectiveness of the remedy.

- **Storage**: Store the remedies in their original containers away from direct light, heat and strong-smelling substances.

- **Overdose**: In case of accidentally taking a number of remedies – do not panic. Taking dozens of tablets is no different to taking just one.

Plant-based Remedies

As with other natural remedies, all different parts of a plant can be used to prepare a homeopathic remedy. In some cases just the roots or leaves are used, in others the whole plant. Each one will be carefully selected to effect symptoms of the disease being treated.

Hypericum *(Hypericum perforatum)*

The St John's wort shrub is native to Asia and Europe, but is now grown worldwide. In homeopathy, the whole fresh plant is used when in flower and it is most commonly given to treat nerve pain following injury, due to its effective action on the central nervous system.

Pain Relief

Hypericum works well on any area affected by nerve pain and injury, but particularly on injuries to the body where there are many nerve endings, such as the spine, head, fingers, toes and lips. It can also help concussion, neuralgia, back pain, pain that shoots upwards, pain after dentistry, small wounds such as bites or splinters, nausea, asthma which worsens in fog, painful piles and rectal nerve pain. In women, late periods accompanied by headaches can also be alleviated.

Aconite

The homeopathic remedy Aconite is made from monk's hood, also known as wolf's bane, and the whole plant is used to prepare the remedy. It is appropriate for conditions that come on suddenly and which are often very acute, sometimes as a result of exposure to cold. Illnesses may follow a fright, particularly in young children.

Treating with Aconite

Conditions that respond to aconite are those characterized by intense pains, such as neuralgia.

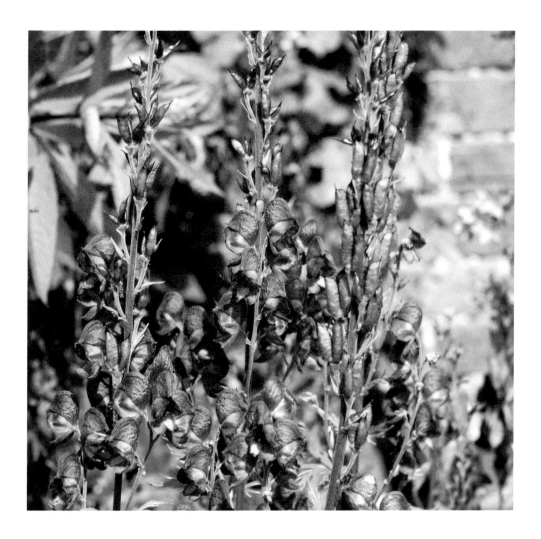

The sufferer cannot bear to be touched and will seem hot and dry with little or no sweat. Violent headaches; inflammation; sudden colds or fevers; a red, raw, sore throat; violent sudden nausea and vomiting, and croupy coughs, particularly those that come on after exposure to cold or dry air, will all respond to Aconite. It can also be used to treat shock and any trauma, either emotional or physical, to which it will respond.

Ipecac *(Ipecacuanha)*

Ipecacuanha is a small, perennial shrub, grown in the tropical rainforests of southern and central America. Homeopathically, the root, collected when the plant is in flower and then dried, is used to treat nausea, vomiting and the accompanying sweats and clamminess. Ipecac is also good for stomach complaints, accompanied by salivating, lack of thirst, weak pulse and fainting, conditions causing breathing difficulties, such as asthma and coughing; coughing and vomiting at the same time. It can also be used to treat persistent nausea.

Drosera *(Drosera rotundifolia)*

The sundew is a carnivorous plant from which the homeopathic remedy drosera is made. Sundew was used in the Middle Ages to treat the plague, and sixteenth-century physicians used it for tuberculosis. Homeopathically, the whole fresh plant is used, mainly to treat coughs and complaints such as whooping cough, characterized by a violent, spasmodic, hollow-sounding cough, triggered by a tickling sensation in the throat. The cough worsens after midnight and at the acute stage is accompanied by retching and vomiting, cold sweats and nosebleeds, after which the patient becomes talkative. This remedy also helps the tingling pain associated with growing pains, stiffness and a hoarse voice.

Gelsemium *(Gelsemium sempervirens)*

The jasmine plant, from which this homeopathic remedy is made, was used as a treatment for fevers in herbalism before being proven in homeopathy. Conditions which affect the nervous system, such as the nerves and muscles, respond well to the remedy. Headaches that worsen with movement or light, muscle pain that accompanies fever, nervous disorders such as multiple sclerosis, nerve inflammation, right-eye pain, heavy, drooping eyelids, inflamed tonsils and summer colds can all be helped. Also fevers, including flushing, an unpleasant taste in the mouth, twitchy muscles and chills. It can help alleviate fears and shock accompanied by shaking or trembling. Visual disturbances and blurred vision can also be treated.

Belladonna *(Atropa)*

The deadly nightshade plant was used in witchcraft during the Middle Ages. Bella donna means 'beautiful woman' in Italian, and women used it in eyedrops to enlarge their pupils, making them more attractive. It is grown throughout Europe and the fresh leaves and flowers are used in homeopathy. Symptoms improve in warmth, standing up, with warm compresses and worsen when cool, on the right side, at 3 p.m., with movement, noise, light, pressure.

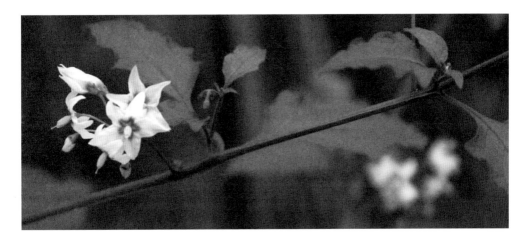

Properties and Uses

- Sudden, intense inflammatory complaints, with flushing and throbbing pains
- For high fevers with staring eyes and dilated pupils
- Calms restless, excitable behaviour
- For wild hallucinations and nightmares
- For instances when the body is very hot with cold feet
- For sensitivity to light and the sun, and touch and movement
- For throbbing headaches
- For earaches, particularly on the right side
- For a bright red tongue and hot dry face

Bryonia *(Bryonia alba)*

Found in central and southern Europe, the deadly root of this plant is bitter-tasting and kills within hours of ingestion. The homeopathic remedy, in which the fresh root is pounded to a pulp, was one of the first to be proved in 1834 by Samuel Hahnemann and is mainly used for conditions that start slowly and worsen with movement.

Uses

It is often used for coughs, colds, headaches and flu that develop slowly and are accompanied by dryness (for instance, in the throat) and great thirst. Bryonia is also useful for joint inflammation such as rheumatism and osteoarthritis, chest and abdominal inflammation, pleurisy, pneumonia, constipation and mastitis. People who need bryonia are like bears with sore heads.

Ruta Grav *(Ruta graveolens)*

Based on the herb rue, which was traditionally used in the sixteenth and seventeenth centuries to prevent the spread of typhus, this homeopathic remedy is useful for bruised bones and tendon injuries, aching bones, deep-aching pain, rheumatism, sciatica, which is worse when lying down and for the restlessness that goes with having to be still or lying down. It is also good for eyestrain, when the eyes feel hot and sore from overuse or reading small print, and accompanying headaches. Other conditions treated include infection after tooth extraction, weak chest with breathing difficulties, prolapsed rectum, constipation with stools that are alternately large and difficult to pass or loose, containing blood and mucus. Symptoms improve with movement, and worsen in the cold and damp, when resting or lying down.

Rhus Tox *(Rhus toxicodendron)*

Poison ivy, or a variety of it, poison oak, is the basis of this homeopathic remedy. Uses include skin complaints characterized by red, itchy, puffy skin that feels like it is burning and which tends to form a scaly surface, such as eczema, herpes, nappy rash, and raised patches of skin

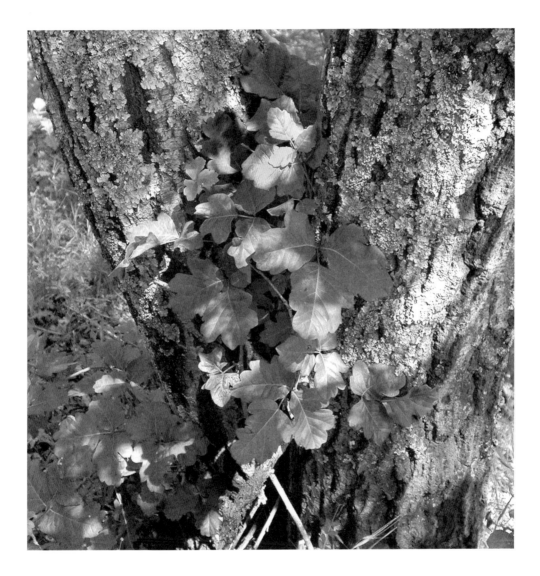

where there is a clear demarcation line between the affected and unaffected part. Muscle and joint pain, such as that associated with rheumatism, osteoarthritis, cramps, restless legs, stiffness in the lower back, numbness in arms and legs and strains can also be alleviated.

Urtica *(Urtica urens)*

The stinging nettle is the basis for this homeopathic remedy. Used both as an internal remedy and external cream, urtica is useful for skin conditions, particularly if the skin is stinging or has the sensation of burning. It is good for rashes, where the skin is blotchy and blistered, such as urticaria (hives) and bee stings, or when there is an allergic reaction, for instance, after eating strawberries. Other conditions alleviated include rheumatism, neuralgia, neuritis, gout, excess uric acid, and in women, vulval itching and painful breasts when there is a block to milk flow. Symptoms improve after massaging the affected area and when lying down, and worsen in cold, damp air, if touched and with water.

Ledum *(Ledum palustre)*

Wild rosemary has been used for its antiseptic qualities for centuries. Homeopathically, ledum is made from the whole fresh plant in flower, which is dried and powdered. Ledum is a useful first-aid remedy and helps prevent infection in cuts and wounds. Complaints that need immediate treatment, such as stings, cuts, grazes, eye injuries and puncture wounds respond well, especially if there is accompanying bruising and the area becomes painful, swollen and puffy. It can also help to alleviate rheumatic pain that starts in the feet and moves up, painful or injured joints which may look pale or bluish and where the affected part feels cold to the touch but the person feels hot.

Lycopodium *(Lycopodium clavatum)*

This plant has long been used to treat stomach complaints and urinary disorders. For homeopathic use the pollen dust is shaken out of the spikes of the fresh plant. This remedy is commonly used to treat digestive complaints, such as vomiting, indigestion, distended abdomen with flatulence, constipation, bleeding piles and hunger which turns to discomfort after eating. Other problems that can be alleviated include swelling in the ankles, feet or hands (oedema); burst blood vessels in the eye; chronic catarrh; psoriasis on the hands and pneumonia.

Symptoms improve when in cool, fresh air, when wearing loose clothing, after hot food and drinks and at night, and are worse on the right side, in stuffy rooms, wearing tight clothing, after overeating or not eating, between 4 a.m. to 8 a.m. and 4 p.m. to 8 p.m.

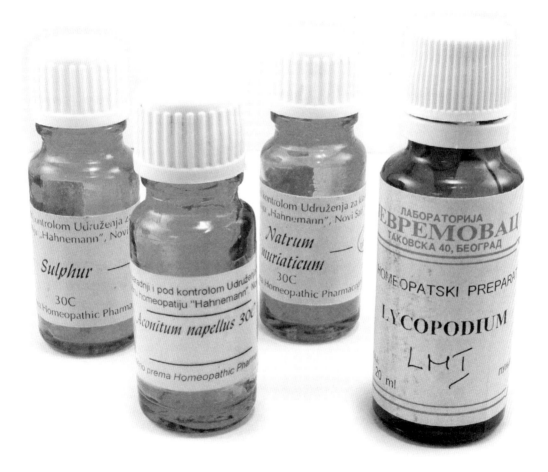

Flower-based Remedies

Flowering plants are a mainstay of homeopathy, and indeed Dr Edward Bach developed a system of 'Flower Remedies' similar to homeopathic remedies, which were said to contain the vibrations of the sun's energy, absorbed by the flower's petals when immersed in sun-warmed water.

Arnica *(Arnica montana)*

Arnica has been used for its healing properties for centuries. It grows in the mountain regions of Europe and Siberia. In folk remedies it was used for aches and bruises and in conventional medicine for rheumatism, gout and dysentery. When in flower the whole fresh plant is used externally as a cream for sprains and bruises, and internally to treat shock, often following an injury.

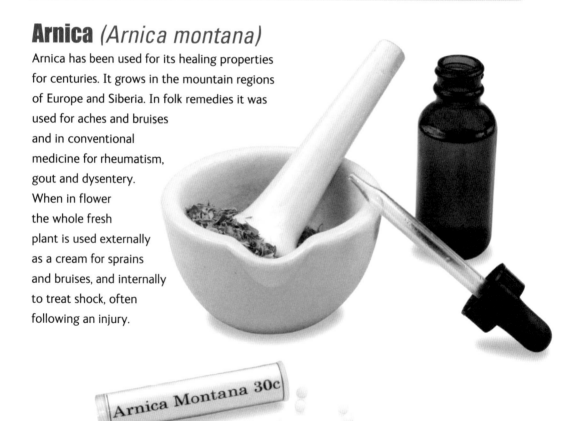

Arnica Montana 30c

External and Internal Uses

Arnica is an effective first-aid treatment for bruising, sprains and strains. Internally, it can help control bleeding and stimulates the healing of damaged tissue. It is also useful for shock, either after an injury or emotional trauma. It can be used for long-term joint and muscle complaints such as osteoarthritis. Internal treatment can aid external conditions such as boils. Remember not to use arnica cream on broken skin.

Chamomilla *(Matricaria recutita)*

Hippocrates was one of the first physicians to understand the medicinal benefits of chamomile. The plant is a member of the daisy family and grows in Europe and America. Homeopathically, the juice is extracted from the whole fresh plant in flower and the remedy is given for those who are sensitive and have a low pain threshold. It is particularly good for children.

Treatment for Sensitive Types

Chamomilla works well for those who are sensitive to pain and are unable to deal with their discomfort, being impatient, rude and angry when ill. Often the reaction seems disproportionate to the amount of pain being felt. Even slight pain may cause sweats and fainting in women and children. Children particularly benefit from the remedy. Teething newborns who are feverish and want to be held all the time, and infants with earache who will not sit still owing to the pain and may scream, can be soothed. Toothache which makes one cheek red and hot can also be alleviated. Other conditions treated include tinnitus, heartburn, heavy, painful periods and diarrhoea with slimy green stools.

Daisy *(Bellis perennis)*

This homeopathic remedy is similar to arnica, hypericum and calendula, and is mainly used following accidents, sprains and bruises. Bellis perennis is known as 'woundwort' or English arnica. It is most appropriate for wounds that are deeper within the body, such as in the abdomen or pelvis. The whole daisy plant is used to make this remedy.

Bellis perennis is best for injuries to the back or slipped discs, after major surgical operations, injuries or blows to the breasts, and where tumours develop from injuries. Helpful after Caesarean section and childbirth, and during pregnancy when there is lower back ache and the uterus feels sore and squeezed.

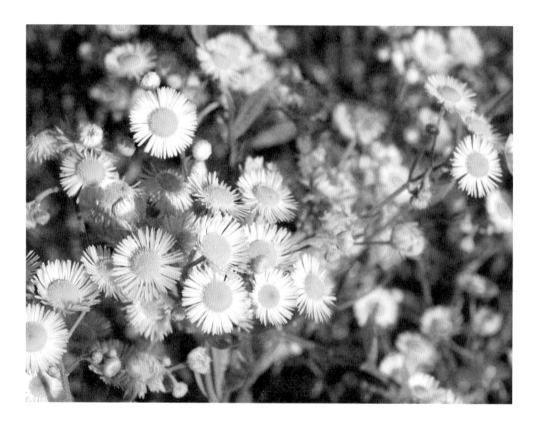

Euphrasia *(Euphrasia officinalis)*

Eyebright – as its name suggests – has been used for centuries to treat eye problems. Homeopathically, the whole fresh plant is used when in flower to make a remedy for sore, irritated eyes and eye injuries.

Easing Inflammation

Euphrasia is useful for any eye irritation or inflammation, such as conjunctivitis, inflammation of the eyelid or iris and small blisters on the cornea. Effective for dimmed vision, dislike of bright lights; watery, irritated eyes associated with hay fever sufferers, but accompanied by only bland nasal discharge; colds accompanied by flushed face and runny catarrh; eye injuries; dry eyes associated with the menopause. Also useful for constipation, exploding headaches, short painful periods, the early stages of measles and, in men, inflammation of the prostate gland.

Colocynth *(Colocynthis)*

The homeopathic remedy colocynth is made from the bitter apple, a fruit that grows in hot, arid conditions. In ancient times, the bitter apple was used by the Greeks as a purgative, to induce abortion and for derangement, dropsy and lethargy. Homeopathically, the fruit is dried and powdered, without the seeds.

It is mainly used to treat symptoms brought on by anger, particularly suppressed anger, such as neuralgia and abdominal pain; stomach pain, facial neuralgia and headaches respond well, as does nerve pain in the ovaries or kidneys; gout, sciatica and rheumatism symptoms can also be helped. Symptoms improve in the warmth, after flatulence or drinking coffee, but worsen after eating, when indignant or angry and in damp, cold weather.

Calendula *(Calendula)*

The common, or pot, marigold has been used for centuries for its healing properties. It is a popular herbal medicine and is used for its anti-inflammatory and anti-microbial qualities in conditions ranging from skin complaints to cancer. As a cream, ointment or tincture it is a common first-aid treatment for cuts, grazes and scalds in both herbal and homeopathic medicine. Homeopathically, the fresh leaves and flowers of the plant are used to make the remedy and a cream for external use.

Clotting Properties

It is well-known for its cleansing antiseptic qualities and to promote healing by aiding clotting. After childbirth, it is often used by midwives in baths or lotions to aid perineal tears. After tooth extraction profuse bleeding can be controlled by gargling with calendula in cooled boiled water.

Ensure cuts are clean before use so that rapid healing does not close in dirt or germs. Do not use for puncture wounds or deep cuts, as rapid healing may seal the infection inside the wound.

Pulsatilla *(Pulsatilla nigricans)*

This homeopathic remedy is made from the pasque flower, or windflower. Pulsatilla can help relieve a number of digestive problems, such as rich food causing lack of sleep; a tight stomach on waking in the morning; bad reactions to rich or fatty food, particularly pork; heaviness under breastbone after eating; cravings for sweet foods and a rumbling stomach.

Women's Problems

In women, lack of periods or late periods, particularly if due to shock or illness, thick, stinging discharge and menopausal problems, all of which tend to be accompanied by crying and depression, can be helped. Moodiness, depression and fears of being alone can also be treated. Ailments characterised by excessive discharge or secretions, such as conjunctivitis, catarrh with yellow phlegm, sinusitis and a runny nose, can also be alleviated. Symptoms improve in fresh air, with gentle movement and with sympathy, and worsen in the heat, after eating rich foods, after lengthy standing, when lying on the left side and in the evening.

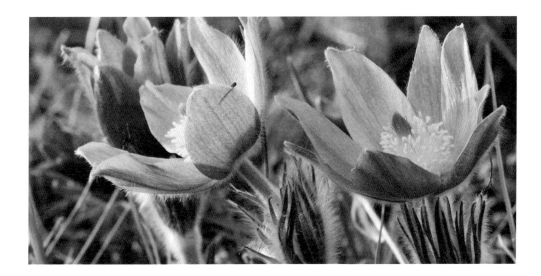

Properties and Uses

- Relieves digestive disorders, gynaecological conditions, emotional traumas
- For people who avoid confrontations
- To treat depression
- For the self-conscious
- For those who cry easily
- For fear of being alone, the dark, insanity and death
- Treats ailments characterized by discharge
- For gynaecological conditions
- For digestive problems
- For a bad taste in the mouth, dry mouth
- Relieves aching joints

Nut- and Seed-based Remedies

The nuts and seeds of plants can be powerful curatives when used homeopathically. The juice from the nuts can be extracted and distilled, or the nuts and seeds can be powdered and then distilled using traditional homeopathic methods.

Anacardium

Grown in the East Indies, the Hindus use the acrid black juice of this nut to burn away moles, warts and other skin complaints. The Arabians used the juice for a number of conditions, such as mental illness, memory loss and paralysis. Homeopathically, cardol – the juice extracted from the pith between the shell and kernel – is used to make the remedy which is prescribed for 'tight' feelings of pain.

Treatment with Anacardium

This remedy is useful when there is a feeling of tightness or constricted pain. Other conditions that may be relieved are itchy skin, piles, constipation, indigestion, duodenal ulcers (which feel better immediately after eating, but cause discomfort two hours later) and rheumatism. It is particularly beneficial for those who suffer from an inferiority complex and who want to prove themselves, or for those who feel that they have been humiliated and want to vent their anger.

Coffea *(Coffea arabica* or *Coffea cruda)*

Coffee is native to Arabia and Ethiopia and is thought to have been first drunk in Persia. Now grown in central America and the West Indies, it has been used widely for medicinal purposes as a diuretic, painkiller and to ease indigestion. It is also a well-known stimulant. Homeopathically, coffea is made from the raw berries of the coffee tree.

Mental Disorders

Commonly used to treat excessive mental activity, when the mind seems to be buzzing and where the person is very excitable and hypersensitive (e.g. toothache or labour pain); when all the senses are so acutely affected that any noise, smell or touch seem unbearable; headaches which are so severe it feels like a nail is being driven into the skull; palpitations when excited or angry; and for acute premenstrual symptoms. Symptoms may appear after exhaustion, trauma or a failed relationship. A high can descend into gloom and despair.

Symptoms

Symptoms improve in the warmth, after lying down and when holding cold water in the mouth, and worsen for extreme emotions such as anger, with touch, smells or noise and in cold, windy weather.

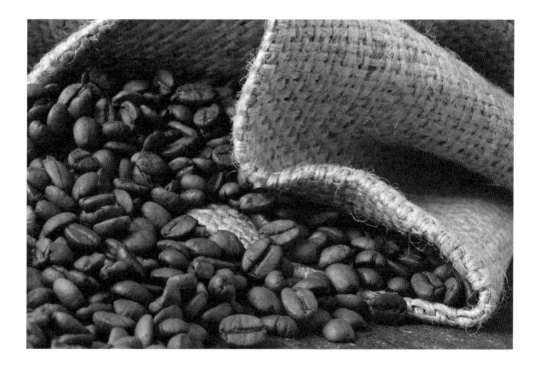

Ignatia *(Ignatia amara)*

The seeds of the *Ignatia amara* tree have been used through the centuries for their healing properties. Homeopathically, the seeds are separated from their pods and powdered. The remedy is used to treat emotional upsets, such as shock and grief, as the strychnine acts on the central nervous system.

Nervous Conditions

Ignatia is commonly used to treat conditions that occur as a result of emotional upheaval. Shock, anger and grief, for instance, over the break-up of a relationship, or suppression of these feelings can be treated, as can bereavement characterized by changes of mood, insomnia and hysteria. Conditions such as nervous headaches, fainting, sweating, choking, or a tickly cough which are a result of emotional upset also respond well. Ailments that are changeable or symptoms that seem contradictory, for instance, a sore throat that feels better after eating solids, are helped. In women, lack of periods or uterine spasms during periods, constipation, piles and shooting pain in a prolapsed rectum are relieved.

Nux Vomica *(Strychnos nux-vomica)*

Made from the poisonous nut plant, which contains strychnine, this remedy is normally used for oversensitivity, irritability and digestive problems. It works well for those who bottle up their anger, who are never satisfied, are prone to arguments, dislike having to depend on others and prefer being left alone. It is also used for conditions such as nausea, vomiting, diarrhoea, indigestion, constipation and piles, which may be brought on by the overindulgence of certain foods or due to suppressing the emotions of mental overwork.

Other Uses

Other problems it can alleviate include flu, retching coughs, colds with a blocked nose at night and runny nose during the day, chills, headaches which are worse due to mental exertion. In women, it helps with erratic, early or heavy periods, morning sickness, constant urination and labour pain. Symptoms improve when lying down and after sleep, in warmth and humidity, in the evening, after washing and with pressure, and worsen in cold, windy weather, in the morning, in open air or under the sun, two hours after food and after mental exhaustion.

China
(China officinalis)

The China remedy is made from Peruvian bark – grown in the tropical rainforests of South America, in India and Southeast Asia – which is stripped and dried. Quinine, an extract of the bark, was the first substance to be tested and proven by Samuel Hahnemann in 1790. He used quinine on himself, noting that large doses caused similar symptoms to malaria, while small doses acted as an antidote. Quinine is still used in conventional medicine today as part of treatment for malaria.

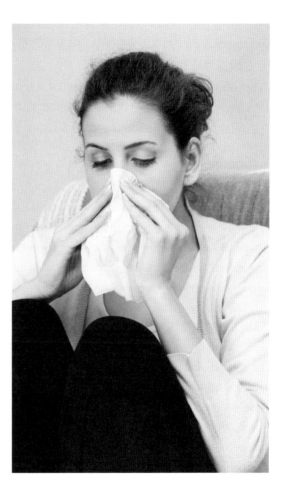

Uses

China aids recovery from nervous exhaustion after debilitating illness and as a result of loss of fluids from vomiting, diarrhoea or sweating. It is also used for digestive conditions such as gastroenteritis, flatulence and gall bladder problems, mental upsets such as lack of concentration, indifference and outbursts that are out of character. Neuralgia, dizziness, tired and twitchy muscles, tinnitus and haemorrhages can also be treated.

Animal-based Remedies

Homeopathy uses a wide range of natural-occurring products, and not all of them are plant-based. Both land and marine animals provide remedies for ailments as diverse as insect bites and hormone imbalance.

Apis *(Apis mellifera)*

The bee is known for its unique ability to produce honey and for its painful sting. In homeopathy, Apis is used to treat stinging pain and inflamed, burning skin which has swollen up and is painful to touch. Found commonly in Europe, Canada and America, the whole live bee is used homeopathically, including its sting, and is dissolved in alcohol. Symptoms improve under cool conditions, but worsen when touched, in heat or during sleep.

Skin Complaints

Apis is used for complaints, such as bites, stings and urticaria, when the skin becomes swollen, red and itchy, or burns and stings, and is sensitive to the touch. It is also used for urinary tract infections, such as cystitis and for urine and fluid retention. Allergic reactions that affect the nose, eyes and throat, including anaphylactic shock, when watery swelling occurs, and complaints in which joints become swollen, such as arthritis, can also be treated. It is also good for fever accompanied by dry skin, a sore throat, severe headache and lack of thirst. During pregnancy, take care to avoid Apis below a 30c potency.

Properties and Uses

 Relieves hot stinging pain, smarting, watery swellings
 Reduces sensitivity to touch
 Lowers fever accompanied by dry skin
 Relieves violent headache

Helps lack of thirst
 Helps scant urination
 Reduces restlessness
 Diminishes jealousy and irritability
 Helps unpredictability

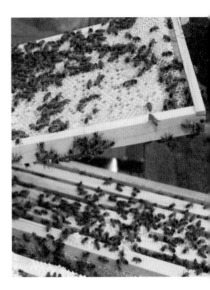

Lachesis *(Trigonocephalus lachesis)*

The South American bushmaster snake, whose venom forms the basis of this homeopathic remedy, is extremely poisonous, and affects the heart and central nervous system. The remedy uses fresh venom and treats wounds that are slow to heal or wounds that bleed profusely.

Blood-related Problems

Lachesis is helpful for premenstrual problems such as erratic pain, relieved by blood flow and problems associated with the menopause, such as hot flushes and dizziness. It works well for any problems connected with blood flow and circulation, such as varicose veins, irregular pulse, angina and palpitations. Problems that occur on the left side, such as earache, headaches and sore throats can be alleviated; wounds that are not healing well, such as bleeding piles, ulcers and cuts are also helped.

Other conditions that can be treated include nervous disorders such as fainting and petit mal epileptic attacks; blue wounds; purplish, bloated face; fever; sweats; pulsations; waking up feeling as if choking and swollen glands.

Symptoms

Symptoms improve after discharges, such as menstruation, nosebleeds or bowel movement, in fresh air and after a cold drink, and are worse on the left side, with sleep, when touched, with motion, in heat, and after hot drinks.

Sepia *(Sepia officinalis)*

Medicinally, cuttlefish ink has historically been used to treat conditions such as kidney stones, hair loss and gonorrhoea. Today, the homeopathic remedy sepia is most commonly used by women and is used to treat complaints such as menstrual problems and hormonal imbalances.

Female Complaints

It is useful for women who feel dragged down both physically and emotionally, as well as for complaints relating to the vagina, ovaries and uterus, such as heavy or painful periods, PMS, menopausal hot flushes, thrush, conditions associated with pregnancy, and the feeling of a sagging abdomen, accompanied by the need to cross the legs. Pain during sex, aversion to sex or exhaustion afterwards can also be treated. Also, any situation where the woman is feeling emotionally and physically tired and lacking in energy. It is also useful for headaches with nausea, hair loss, dizziness, offensive sweating, indigestion, skin discoloration and circulatory problems.

The Sepia Type

The sepia type tends to be female, tall, dark and with sallow skin. They are dignified and attractive, love dancing, but tend to be detached emotionally, often playing the martyr role. They have strong opinions, hating to be contradicted, and are often resentful of responsibilities. Children tend to be sallow, sweaty-skinned, tire easily; are sensitive to weather; moody and negative, dislike being left alone and parties; and have a tendency to constipation.

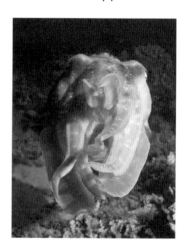

Spongia *(Spongia tosta)*

Sponge was first noted for its medicinal purposes more than 600 years ago, when it was used as a treatment for goitre, the swelling of the thyroid gland, which is brought on by a deficiency in iodine. The homeopathic remedy spongia works particularly well for children's croup, characterized by sneezing and a hoarse, dry barking cough, with the patient waking in alarm with the feeling of suffocation, later followed by thick mucus which is difficult to bring up. Associated symptoms of coughs, such as hoarseness, dryness of the larynx from a cold, headaches which are worse when lying down, but improve when sitting up, bronchitis, dry mucous membranes and feeling heavy and exhausted are also helped. Laryngitis, where the throat is raw and dry and feels like it is burning, responds well. It is also good if chest conditions or tuberculosis run in the family.

Symptoms of the Spongia Type

Symptoms improve with warm food and drinks and when sitting up, and worsen when talking, swallowing, eating sweet food or cold drinks, moving, touching the affected area, lying with the head lower than the feet and around midnight.

Cantharis *(Lytta vesicatoria* or *Cantharis vesicatoria)*

The homeopathic remedy cantharis is made from Spanish fly, a bright green beetle that is native to southern Europe and western Asia. It emits a rapid-acting irritant, cantharidin, causing blistering, hence its other common name ('cantharides' or 'cantharis'), despite actually being from the *Meloidae* family as opposed to the *Cantharidae* family.

Ailments treated are those characterized by burning or stinging, particularly urinary tract infections such as cystitis with frequent but painful urination, insect bites, burns and scalds, infections, burning abdominal pains and stinging diarrhoea. It is also for infections that spread rapidly or conditions that quickly deteriorate. Mental problems such as rage, agitation leading to violence, excessive sexual desire and severe anxiety can be relieved. Symptoms improve in the warmth, with massage, after flatulence or burping and at night, and worsen with movement, after drinking coffee or cold water and in the afternoon.

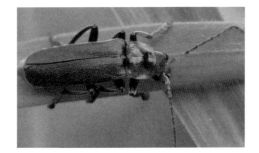

Biochemic Tissue Salts

Biochemic tissue salts are homeopathically prepared and were introduced at the end of the nineteenth century by a German doctor, Wilhelm Schüssler. He believed that many diseases were caused by a deficiency of one or more of 12 vital minerals, which would manifest as particular symptoms. An imbalance in these salts would also cause a range of illnesses. Replacing them in small, easily absorbed doses restores balance and allows the body to heal itself.

Calc Fluor *(Calcarea fluorica)*

Calc Fluor is used homeopathically and mainly in pregnancy. It can improve the elasticity in the skin, veins or glands. As a tissue salt it helps with piles, varicose veins, cold sores, cracked tongues and lips. Physical symptoms relieved include inflamed skin and stretch marks in pregnancy, swollen glands, and enamel deficiency of teeth.

Calc Phos *(Calcarea phosphorica)*

Calcium phosphate is a mineral salt which is the main constituent – along with collagen – of bones and teeth. A natural version is the mineral apatite. For homeopathic use, it is prepared chemically from dilute phosphoric acid and calcium hydroxide, which form fine particles of calcium phosphate. These are then filtered and dried. The remedy is also used as a tissue salt and used to treat bone and teeth complaints.

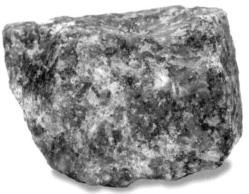

Calc Phos Treatment

Used to treat slow growth and growing pains in children, for instance, when the fontanelles are slow to close in an infant, painful teething and numbness, and tingling attributed to growing. It is also used to treat bones that are healing slowly. Slow recovery after illness due to weakness and fatigue, digestive problems such as diarrhoea and indigestion and recurrent throat infections can be helped.

Ferrum Phos *(Ferrum phosphoricum)*

The Ferrum Phos remedy is made from iron phosphate, a chemical combination of iron sulphate, sodium phosphate and sodium acetate. It has a variety of different uses, including the first stages of inflammation or infection, when more blood is flowing to the affected areas, causing congestion before the onset of other symptoms.

Other Uses

Ferrum Phos is also good for slow-starting colds accompanied by nosebleeds; fevers, accompanied by hacking coughs; headaches that are helped by cool water; rheumatic pain; gastritis including vomiting undigested food; indigestion with sour-tasting burps; haemorrhages in women; intermittent, painful, periods; stress incontinence; and the first stages of dysentery with bloody stools.

Kali Mur *(Kali muriaticum)*

This remedy works very well in a low potency in acute situations. It is good for earache with blocked Eustachian tubes, and for indigestion and diarrhoea caused by too much rich and fatty food. It is also helpful in the secondary stages of inflammatory complaints.

Properties and Uses

 For thick white discharges
 For ulcerated throat

Unblocks sinuses
 Alleviates dark menstrual flow
 Alleviates constipation
 Soothes blister-like eruptions

Kali Phos *(Kali phosphoricum)*

Homeopathically, Kali Phos is prepared by adding dilute phosphoric acid to a solution of potassium carbonate (also known as potash). Used to treat mental and physical exhaustion, particularly when the nerves become so frayed the patient is on edge and sensitive to any disturbance or distraction. Sufferers usually wish to be left alone and become introverted. Conditions such as sensitivity to cold, pus or yellow vaginal discharge, discharge from the lungs or in the stools, muscle fatigue, early morning awakening and chronic fatigue syndrome can all be alleviated.

Mag Phos *(Magnesia phosphorica)*

The Mag Phos homeopathic remedy is made chemically from magnesium sulphate and sodium phosphate, and has an antispasmodic effect. It is a useful remedy for any type of cramp, from infant colic and abdominal cramp to menstrual pains and writer's cramp, with the sufferer doubled up in pain. Abdominal cramps are sharp and intense, with the pain jumping from one part to another and may improve when bending, with heat and hard pressure and worsen in the cold, draughts and at night. Headaches and neuralgia, when the head throbs, the face is flushed and pain suddenly comes and goes, improves in the warmth and if the head is bound. Symptoms worsen in the cold, in draughty conditions and at night. Pains tend to be on the right side of the body.

Nat Mur *(Natrum muriaticum)*

Homeopathically, the Nat Mur remedy is made from rock salt, which is formed through the evaporation of salty water, leaving a crusty crystalline solid. The remedy is used to treat a number of conditions, from emotional problems to ailments characterized by a discharge.

Nat Mur Treatments

Nat Mur works well on emotional problems such as distress, restlessness and depression, which tend to occur because of the suppression of other emotions, such as fear and grief. Conditions characterized by secretions or discharge, such as colds, catarrh, vaginismus, mouth ulcers, nasal boils, acne and cold sores, and other skin complaints such as hangnails, warts and a cracked lower lip are alleviated. In women, it helps with erratic periods, periods which have stopped due to stress, shock or grief, malaise, swollen ankles before and after a period, and for a dry or sore vagina. Headaches, caused by trauma or exercise; explosive headaches or blinding migraines also respond well.

Silica

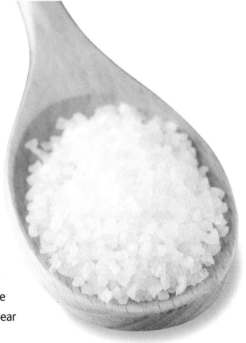

Also called silicea, this homeopathic remedy is prepared from silicon dioxide. It is good for complaints that have occurred as a result of low immunity due to undernourishment, such as colds, ear infections and catarrh. Also for skin and bone conditions, such as acne, weak nails, slow growth or fontanelles that are slow to close in babies, slow-healing fractures, expelling splinters, glass shards or thorns from body tissue, problems associated with the nervous system, such as colic and migraines. Other problems alleviated include catarrh with thick, yellow discharge, enlarged lymph nodes, offensive sweat, headaches which start at the back of the head and move over the forehead, glue ear and restless sleep.

Mineral-based Remedies

In addition to the 12 biochemic tissue salts, there are many other minerals used to prepare homeopathic remedies. Some minerals are important for our bodies to function efficiently and should be part of a balanced diet, but distillations of some can also be used to treat a variety of ailments.

Sulphur *(Sulphur brimstone)*

This homeopathic remedy is extracted from the mineral and can be used to treat digestive and skin disorders. It is useful for hot, red, itchy skin associated with problems such as eczema and nappy rash, digestive complaints such as vomiting and diarrhoea that occur in the morning, indigestion which is made worse by drinking milk, and hunger pangs.

Other Uses

It can also treat offensive odours, such as foul-smelling sweat or discharge, premenstrual symptoms such as irritability and headaches and menopausal symptoms, such as flushing and dizzy spells. It is also useful if another remedy has not worked, or if the picture remedy is not clear. Other problems, such as lack of energy, restless sleep, depression, fever, burning pains and eruptions, congestions and back pain can also be helped.

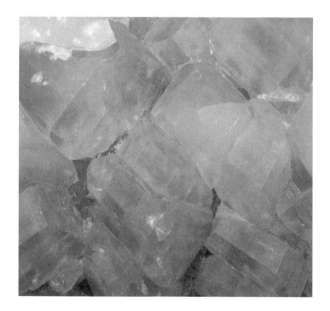

Symptoms

Symptoms improve when lying on the right side in warm, dry, fresh air, after physical activity, and worsen in stuffy atmospheres, in the morning, particularly around 11 a.m. and at night, in the damp and cold, and after washing.

Phosphorus

Our bodies need phosphorus for the healthy functioning of our teeth, bones, bodily fluids and deoxyribonucleic acid (DNA). In conventional medicine it has been used to treat conditions as diverse as measles and malaria. Homeopathically, it is mainly given to those suffering from anxiety and digestive disorders.

Nervous and Digestive Conditions

Phosphorus is used to treat symptoms such as exhaustion, insomnia, nerves that are caused by underlying stress, anxiety and fears, for instance, due to exam pressure, overwork or fears of dying.

Other problems that can be helped include digestive problems such as nausea and vomiting due to coughing, stress or food poisoning; cravings for certain foods and pressure in the stomach; symptoms of poor circulation such as cold or overheated fingers and toes; excessive bleeding, such as bleeding gums, nosebleeds and heavy periods; respiratory problems such as acute bronchitis or asthma; difficulty in breathing; tight chest; pneumonia; dry, tickly coughs and red-tinged phlegm.

Symptoms

Symptoms improve in fresh air, after sleeping, when touched and when lying on the right side, and worsen in the morning and evenings, after mental or physical exertion, after hot food or drinks, when lying on the left side and in thunderstorms.

Arsenic *(Arsenicum album)*

Arsenic has a rather questionable reputation as a murder weapon. Indeed, poisoning by arsenic is the mainstay of many murder mysteries. Thankfully, arsenic poisoning is no longer a common cause of death. In the past, small doses were given to treat syphilis, anthrax and to improve stamina. Arsenic is made of metallic crystals which cannot be destroyed. In homeopathy, a minute compound of arsenic is used, which works beneficially on the sensitive lining of the digestive tract and respiratory system.

Arsenic Treatment

Arsenicum album is given to those suffering from anxiety, being alone, fear of the dark, fear of failure, which are caused by underlying feelings of insecurity. It is also useful for problems of the digestive system, such as indigestion, diarrhoea and vomiting, food poisoning and excessive eating, such as over-consumption of fruit or ice cream and drinking too much alcohol.

Arsenic can be used to treat a range of conditions which particularly sting or burn, such as mouth ulcers, sore lips, eye inflammation, vomiting and burning pains in the rectum. Asthma, fatigue, fluid retention, especially around the ankles, can also be helped.

Ant Crud *(Antimonium crudum)*

This homeopathic remedy is prepared from black sulphide of antimony, which occurs naturally as an ore. It is known as the 'pig's remedy', because it is most appropriate for those with a large appetite, and when the stomach and digestive system are affected.

Properties and Uses

Ant Crud is useful for treating an upset stomach and vomiting caused by overeating. Vomit is normally acidic. Children who will benefit from Ant Crud may be irritable and fretful, but will not want attention. In low dosages, Ant Crud can be taken for long periods of time to treat calluses and corns on the feet. It is also useful for:

- ✔ Irritability and fretfulness
- ✔ Treating a thick white coating on the tongue
- ✔ Lumpy discharge
- ✔ Rough, hardened, cracked skin
- ✔ Nostrils, corners of the mouth and sore, cracked feet
- ✔ Sensitive feet
- ✔ Sensitivity to cold

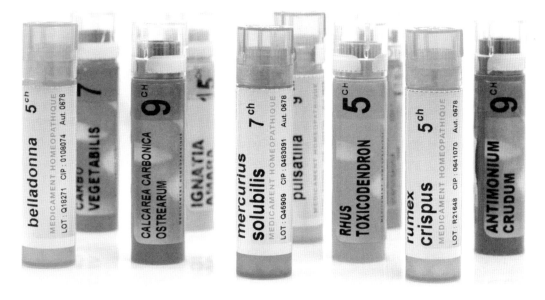

Ant Tart *(Antimonium Tartaricum)*

Antimony potassium tartrate is a poisonous crystalline salt that has no colour or odour and is used as a fix for leather, textiles and in insecticides. In the past, it was used in conventional medicine as an emetic for internal worms, to induce vomiting and as an expectorant. Homeopathically, it is used to treat gastric disorders and chest complaints. Symptoms improve when sitting up, after vomiting and in cold air; they worsen in stuffy rooms and, if wearing too much, with movement or when lying down.

Properties and Uses

Antimonium tart can be used for the following ailments:

- **For people who are irritable, anxious and despairing**
- **For chest complaints and coughs with rattling breathing and great difficulty in bringing up phlegm**
- **For stomach upsets with nausea, weakness and cold sweats**
- **For people who are uninterested in food and drink**
- **To treat drowsiness**

Calc Carb *(Calcarea carbonica)*

This homeopathic remedy is derived from the mother-of-pearl in oyster shells. This remedy is most often used to help problems relating to the teeth and bones. It is used to treat bones and joints which are slow to develop or slow to heal after injury and relieves complaints that may be due to this, such as backache. It also helps slow-growing teeth and pain during teething. Right-sided headaches, premenstrual tension, heavy periods, menopause problems, thrush, eczema, arthritis, asthma and digestive problems can also be helped.

Merc Sol *(Mercurius solubilis)*

In Roman mythology, Mercury was the messenger of the gods. In recent centuries, the substance has been used for various medicinal purposes.

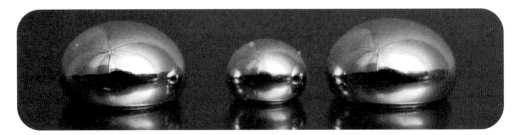

Merc Sol Treatment

Conditions characterized by a smelly discharge are helped by this remedy, including chronic conjunctivitis, pus secretions from the ears, watery catarrh, nasal cold sores, glutinous saliva that stains the pillow during sleep, throat ulcers which make swallowing painful, phlegmy coughs that worsen in the warmth and at night, drenching sweats, pus-filled skin eruptions, sores, and in women, excessive vaginal discharge and green-looking stools flecked with blood. In the mouth and throat, gingivitis, thrush, bad breath, loose teeth in infected gums, swollen tonsils and ulcers can be helped.

Hepar Sulph *(Hepar sulphuris)*

This homeopathic remedy is made from heating the calcareous inner layer of oyster shells with flowers of sulphur, and is used to treat skin infections and ailments accompanied by a discharge. Symptoms improve in warmth, after applying warm compresses and after eating, and worsen in the morning, in the cold, when touching or lying on the affected parts.

The Hepar Sulph Type

Ailments that respond well to hepar sulph include conjunctivitis, sinusitis, cold sores and mouth ulcers, as well as general infections such as earache, tonsillitis, phlegm-filled chests and flu. It is also used for infections to aid expelling pus, such as acne, where the spots are sensitive to touch. Other conditions helped include colds accompanied by a tickly cough and dry, hoarse coughs accompanied by phlegm.

Arg Nit *(Argentum nitricum)*

Silver nitrate, the source of this remedy, was given the names 'Hell Stone' or 'Devil's Stone' because of its corrosive effect. Silver nitrate is extracted from the mineral acanthite, the main ore of silver. Safe in small doses, large amounts are poisonous, causing breathing problems and damaging the kidneys, liver, spleen and aorta, and overdosing affects the skin, turning it permanently blue. In homeopathy, the remedy is most frequently used for nervous and digestive complaints.

Anxiety-related Conditions

Arg Nit is mainly used for fear and anxiety, usually brought on by stress, and can help problems, such as claustrophobia, dangerous impulses and stage fright. It can also control the overwhelming feeling that something awful is about to happen. It is very useful for digestive problems, such as diarrhoea and vomiting, particularly if the symptoms are brought on by nerves and headaches that begin slowly and are caused by overeating sweet foods. It also helps other conditions such as asthma, colic in babies, epilepsy, warts and sore throats. During labour, it can help bring relief when bearing down.

Kali Bich *(Kali bichromicum)*

This homeopathic remedy is useful for any condition that affects the mucous membranes, leading to a stringy, yellow or white discharge. It can help alleviate problems such as sinusitis, glue ear, coughs and colds accompanied by catarrh or where the affected areas feel congested and under pressure. Vomiting, where the cause is a digestive disorder and yellow mucus is ejected, can also be helped, as can rheumatic pain in joints when the pain tends to move about and becomes worse in hot weather. Migraines that begin at night, feel worse when bending, but get better when pressure is applied to the base of the nose can also be treated with kali bich.

Kali Carb *(Kali carbonicum)*

This remedy is used when the potassium/sodium balance of the body is upset. Stabbing pains are an indication that this imbalance is present. It is useful for catarrhal, congestive headaches, dry coughs with some phlegm which become worse after eating and drinking. It also good for chronic bronchitis, wheeziness and flatulence.

Properties and Uses

 Reduces sensitivity to draught or movement
 Alleviates stitching pains

For dry hacking, barking coughs, particularly in cold air

 For swelling between eyelids and eyebrows

Causticum *(Causticum hahnemanni)*

This remedy was invented and proved by Samuel Hahnemann and is unique to homeopathy. It is made chemically from quicklime (calcium oxide) and potassium bisulphate. Hahnemann found that it caused a burning taste in the back of the mouth and an acerbic sensation. It is used for a set of symptoms known as the causticum cough and for neuromuscular conditions.

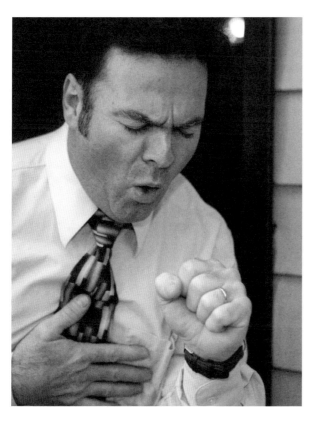

The Causticum Cough

Symptoms of the causticum cough include a raw, throat with a dry, tickly cough; a hard, racking cough; chest filled with mucus which is difficult to cough up; incontinence with the cough and coughing that is worse on breathing out. It also helps neuromuscular problems such as weakness, stiffness, neuralgia, tearing pains in the joints, muscles and bones, cramps, particularly affecting the vocal chords, bladder, larynx or right side of the face. Other conditions alleviated include dizziness when bending forward, heartburn in pregnancy, burning rheumatic pain, roaring in the ears, nasal soreness and tender scars.

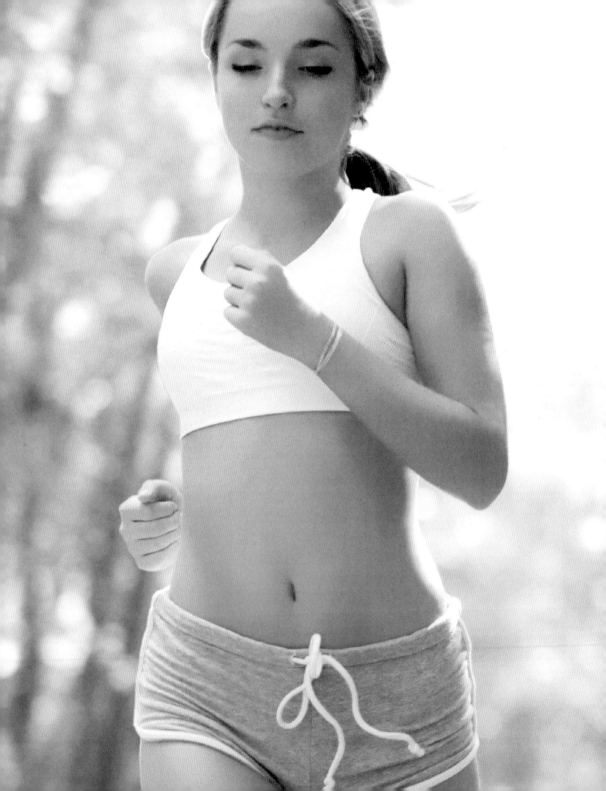

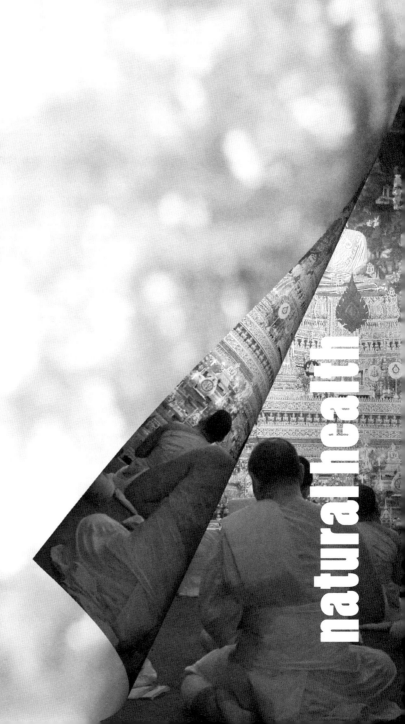

natural health

Understanding Naturopathy

Originally coined by the German pioneer Benedict Lust, naturopathy literally means 'natural treatment', and today its practitioners are generally those trained at specialist colleges in a range of skills that include acupuncture, herbalism, homeopathy, osteopathy, hydrotherapy, massage, nutrition and diet.

Components for Good Health

Naturopaths believe that four basic components make up good health: clean air, clean water, clean food from good earth, exercise and healthy living. All naturopathic treatments work with some of these elements – and often all of them – to restore health and vitality. Naturopaths believe that infections seldom occur if the body is looked after the way nature intended, and that the body will cure itself of anything as long as it takes in only pure air and water, is kept clean, given the right food and undertakes healthy activity.

Illness and Cure

However, naturopaths also believe that getting ill is natural and that methods of cure should follow the same natural principles. So, far from being suppressed, symptoms of illness should be encouraged to come out and the body helped and encouraged to fight back and find its proper balance – or homestastis – again. Naturopaths will routinely encourage brief fasting to get over simple infections such as flu and also address the health of the bowels, where important nutrients are absorbed by the bloodstream.

Most naturopaths encourage special diets to clear the gut and eliminate the overgrowth of 'unfriendly' bacteria that can colonize the intestines and contribute to toxicity, allergy and poor immunity. Some naturopaths even make use of a colonic irrigation for washing the gut clean.

The Principles of Naturopathy

Naturopaths follow three main principles when prescribing any treatment:

 Healing: They believe that the body has the power to heal itself, so treatment should not be given to alleviate symptoms but to support the self-healing mechanism (the body's vital force).

 Symptoms: The symptoms of disease are not part of the disease itself but a sign that the body is striving to eliminate toxins and return to its natural state of balance.

 Physical and mental health: As well as being as natural and gentle as possible, all treatments should take into account the mental, emotional and social aspects of a person, as well as the physical.

Guidance for Life

Naturopathy is a philosophy for life rather than a set of inflexible principles. Naturopaths aim to prevent and treat the causes of disease by a system of detailed diagnosis and a wide range of treatments, many of which must be integrated into your lifestyle in order to achieve lasting good health.

The Power of Naturopathy

Naturopathy can help with a wide range of acute and chronic problems, such as anaemia, allergies, arthritis, bronchitis, candida, circulation disorders, constipation, cystitis, eczema and other skin diseases, hangovers, irritable bowel syndrome, migraine, panic attacks, premenstrual syndrome, sinusitis, ulcers and varicose veins. In the case of life-threatening diseases it can improve resistance to infection so there is less risk of complications.

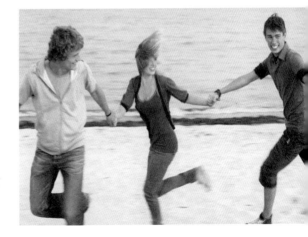

Body Basics

Natural practitioners address each case on an individual basis. On the basis of a full physical and emotional assessment, you will be given treatment that works to balance your body's vital force, or energy. Natural medicine is holistic, which means that it takes into consideration your mind, body and spirit, not just the physical symptoms of disease that present themselves when you are ill.

Disease

Disease is, literally, a state of 'dis-ease', when the body is unbalanced and its systems are not working in harmony. One of the main differences between conventional and natural medicine is the approach to health. Conventional practitioners treat illness as a biological or chemical malfunction of the body. The main premise of conventional medicine is that curing disease will lead to good health, ignoring the fact that pathology is individual to the sufferer, and that each one of us is unique. For example, tonsillitis would be treated with antibiotics in most cases; asthma with Ventolin, steroids or the equivalent; eczema with hydrocortisone cream or another suppressive remedy.

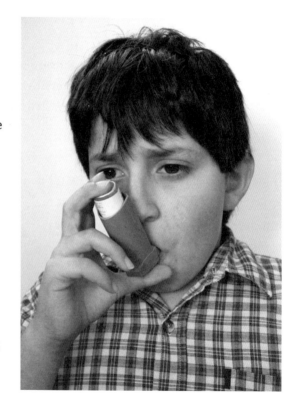

Redressing the Body's Balance

There are well-known physical processes that keep our bodies alive, including the immune system, the brain and nervous system and the endocrine system. These are important on a physical level, and are crucial to maintaining the body's equilibrium. However, they are not the only level of functioning. Equally important is the guiding mechanism. Some complementary medical disciplines believe that energy flows through our bodies, and that illness or 'dis-ease' is caused by blockages and imbalance. Others believe that it is simply a governing force that can be weakened by environmental factors (diet, trauma, stress, pollution, or lack of sleep, for example), so that it can no longer keep the whole body (that is, mind, body and spirit) balanced.

Stress

Stress comes in many forms, and it can be fairly safely described as anything that places undue pressure on the mind, body or spirit. Stress can come from obvious sources: divorce, bereavement, financial problems, over-scheduling, inadequate relaxation and moving house. It can also stem from anything that causes the body to work harder, including a poor diet, inadequate sleep or exercise, constant noise, pollution, chemicals in food and the environment and even injury.

Symptoms of stress include:

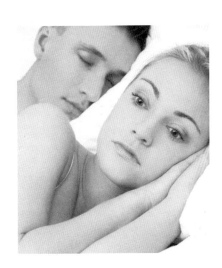

- **Increased breathing and heart rate**
- **Nausea**
- **Tense muscles**
- **Inability to relax**
- 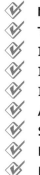 **Irritability (including temper tantrums)**
- **Insomnia**
- **Allergies**
- **Skin problems**
- **Headaches**
- **Fatigue**

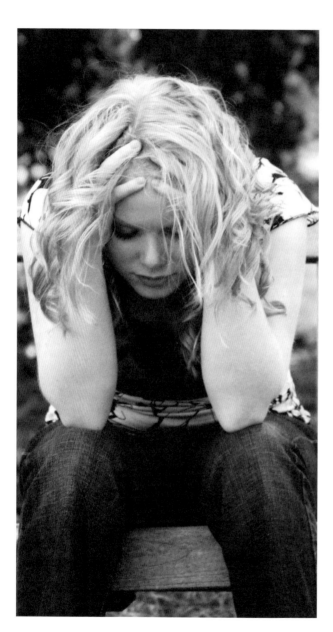

Stages of Stress

All stress factors have an effect on our body, causing it to make a series of rapid physiological changes – called adaptive responses – to deal with threatening or demanding situations. In the first stage of stress, hormones are poured into the bloodstream. The pulse quickens, the lungs take in more oxygen to fuel the muscles, blood sugar increases to supply added energy, digestion slows, and perspiration increases.

In the second stage of stress, the body begins to repair the damage caused by the first stage. If the stressful situation is resolved, the stress symptoms vanish. If the stressful situation continues, however, a third stage, exhaustion, sets in, and the body's energy wears out. This stage may continue until vital organs are affected, and then disease or even death can result.

Immunity

The body has an impressive array of defences to block, trap and kill outside organisms it considers a threat – with a memory to prevent them attacking again. Without this defence system (known as the immune system) most people would constantly fall ill from the wide range of threats to the body.

How the Immune System Works

The immune system consists of the blood supply, the lymph system, and small sets of organs known as the tonsils, thymus gland, and the spleen. Defence against disease is essentially a function of white cells in the blood (leukocytes), and it is one of the jobs of this group of organs to produce these cells.

The immune system is the physical defence mechanism of the body. It is important that it is working at optimum level to protect from infections and infestations, and to ensure quick and efficient recovery when you do succumb to illness.

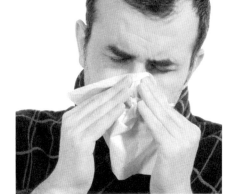

Signs of a weakened immune system include:

- **Fatigue**
- **Listlessness**
- **Repeated infections**
- **Inflammation**
- **Allergic reactions**
- **Slow wound healing**
- **Chronic diarrhoea**

Boosting Immunity Through Naturopathy

The immune system and, indeed, every other system in your body, works more effectively when external factors are under control. The majority of natural remedies and therapies are designed to boost immunity, and even the healthiest of us will benefit from their prudent use.

The idea is not to work on immunity when you become ill, but to ensure that your immune system is strong and healthy enough to resist illness, and to fight it off quickly when you do become ill. This is one of the most important aspects of preventative medicine, which is the cornerstone of the natural health revolution.

Vaccination

Immunization prepares our bodies to fight diseases with which we may come into contact in the future. Immunization against polio, for example, stimulates the immune system to produce antibodies against the polio virus. These antibodies recognize the disease if and when it enters the body at a later date and are ready to fight it.

Some types of immunization, such as those that work against polio, measles, mumps and rubella and against diphtheria, pertussis and tetanus (DTP), are aimed at the general population, primarily at young children. Others are intended for specific people, such as those exposed to dangerous infections during local outbreaks. In many countries, including the US (but not the UK), immunization against certain infections is a requirement for entry to school.

The Value of Vaccinations

There are, however, a number of studies that show how vaccination disrupts normal immune function. When we contract an illness naturally, our bodies begin to build up defences long before symptoms become evident. An illness has to get past the skin, sneezing reflexes, respiratory secretions (mucus), tears, fever, intestinal flora and other elements of immunity before it can gain access to major organs and tissues of the body. As it passes these sites, immunity is built up against the invader. The disease itself is the peak of the 'antibody response'. In other words, symptoms are an indication that our bodies are fighting off the disease.

A child who gets measles, for example, will have 100 per cent immunity to the disease, and the infection will have prepared him or her to respond even more promptly and effectively to other infections acquired in the future.

When the vaccine viruses are injected or squirted directly into the child's body, they bypass the normal immune system response. In other words, it is a fairly serious shock to the body to find itself with a virus at hand, and none of its immune responses prepared.

The Risks of Immunization

By introducing viruses directly into the bloodstream, far from preventing diseases, it actually pushes the disease into a chronic form and deeper into the body, where it then attacks vital organs. It has been suggested that suppressing measles and other infectious diseases in this manner may lead to cancer and other chronic and auto-immune diseases. Despite government assurances to the contrary, there are protesters who are concerned by the link between bowel disorders, encephalitis, epilepsy, MS, diabetes and autism and immunization.

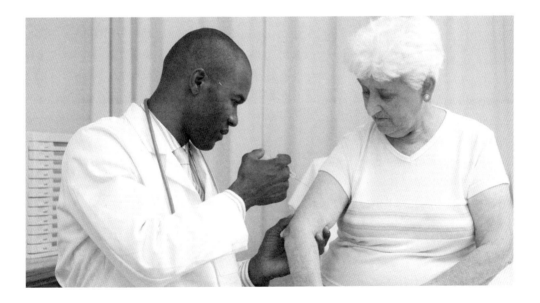

Many natural health practitioners are against the idea of vaccination for all of these reasons. There are homeopathic alternatives available that can be taken instead of vaccinating, but of course this is a very personal choice that must be thought about carefully.

Natural Healing

When you visit a natural health practitioner you will be expected to give details of everything about you and your health in order for your therapist to make an informed decision about treatment. Your symptoms will not be treated, rather, their root cause will be investigated and dealt with.

The Importance of Spirit

Many of us have an instinctive understanding of spirit, a sense of our own life force and being. We may be sensitive to the energy of others and aware of the impact of our own energy. As parents, we can witness the impact of negative energy on our children – a baby becomes anxious and cries when his mother is distressed; a child throws a temper tantrum when his father is rushed and under pressure.

Internal Energy

Spirit is a kind of life energy. Some people call it a soul or 'the spirit', but you do not have to be religious to understand the concept that there is a unique and conscious entity that inhabits and animates the human form. Spirit is seen in terms of love and light and peace. It involves a fundamental personal belief and power, which affects the way you live your life on a daily basis. Spirit is what makes you an individual, and it is something that we all share.

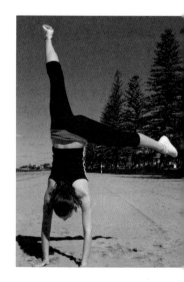

Spirit is an essential element in holistic therapies, and as important as physical and emotional health. So not only will therapists take into consideration the health of your spirit when diagnosing and treating, but they will aim to balance your health on all levels so that you become more in touch with spirit.

Mind, Body and Spirit

Natural practitioners believe that there is something more afoot than simply a physical diagnosis of disease. Indeed, the many elements of health – the mind, body and spirit – are taken into consideration when treating children suffering from virtually any health condition, at any level.

Different therapies and disciplines have a variety of names for the life force: spirit or energy, for example. But the concept remains the same. It is the body's controlling energy. It vitalizes the physical body, and it is the link between the body, soul and mind. The vital force is not a material substance, such as water or air, but it is equally indispensable for life. Its presence distinguishes living things from inanimate matter. When illness occurs, it appears first as a disturbance in this natural energy long before it manifests itself as physical symptoms. This is why we appear grumpy, tired or out of sorts for some time before symptoms actually appear.

The Vital Force

Many of the most ancient therapies are based on the existence of a vital energy flow. Western medicine was, until fairly recently, in agreement that there is an animating force, but as the focus became more scientific, the idea of a vital energy was largely dispensed with. However, the huge wealth of material amassed by scientists into the functioning of the human body is all true and correct, and they do not by any means contradict the idea of the vital force. Physical and chemical mechanisms are merely tools of the vital force, which act upon the physical plane of the body.

Natural remedies work on energy level, focusing our energy and vitality towards healing so that we overcome the problem naturally. They do not heal, in the same way that we might expect if we took a conventional drug, and they do not pretend to do so. Instead, natural remedies encourage the body to heal itself, by operating on a level that is above the physical.

Healing

Healing, also known as spiritual healing, is the channelling of healing energy from its spiritual source to someone who needs it. The channel is usually a person whom we call a healer and the healing energy is usually transferred to the patient through the hands of the healer. The important distinction here is that healing does not come *from* the healer, but *through* him. The word spiritual does not refer to belief in any organized religion, rather it refers to the divine nature of the energy, which healers agree comes from one external, invisible, intelligent source. The healing energy from this source is available to everyone, irrespective of their religious beliefs.

The Root of Illness

Healers see the body, mind and spirit as one interdependent unit and believe all three must work in harmony to maintain health. A problem at any level, be it a broken leg or a feeling of hopelessness, needs healing to restore the balance of the whole person. Sickness often begins in the mind or at the deeper level of the spirit and it is often here that healing begins.

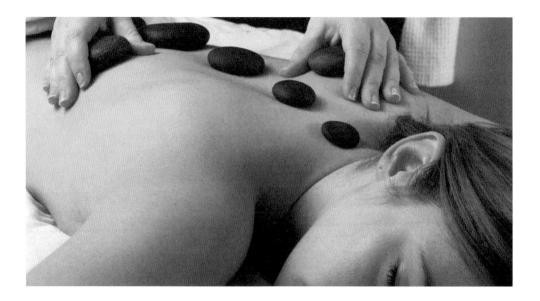

Channelling Energy

When a healer lays his hand on you, he acts as a conductor or channel for the healing energy which he believes has the 'intelligence' to go where it is needed. Healers say that we all have the power to heal, if we choose to develop it. They claim the motivating force behind all healing is unconditional love and the only requirement is that the healer is open to receiving and channelling healing energy. However, some people do seem to have a gift for healing.

Curing Disease

The aim of all medicine, whether conventional or natural, is to effect a cure. Natural therapists claim that the conventional medical system has become obsessed with treating, and in many cases, suppressing and masking symptoms, rather than looking to cure the cause of a problem.

The Law of Cure

Many natural therapies have a rigorous set of principles and systems set up to define a health problem and then to cure it. In homeopathy, for example, the 'law of cure' was developed to pinpoint the steps of the healing process, to ensure that cure was eventually attained. They are:

- **Externalization:** The body seeks to externalize disease – keeping it to more external locations.

- **Progress:** Healing progresses from more important organs to less important ones.

- **Order:** Symptoms should disappear in reverse order to their original appearance.

- **Top down:** Healing progresses from the top of the body downwards (especially in the case of skin rashes).

- **Evaluating success:** You can use this law to help you evaluate the success of any form of treatment you are receiving.

Diet and Exercise

Diet and exercise are a crucial part of overall health and well-being, and are therefore an important aspect of a healthy lifestyle. All natural therapists will encourage moderate exercise and a balanced diet.

Benefits of Exercise

There are many benefits to exercise. Among the most obvious are that it strengthens the cardiovascular system and increases heart mass. It dilates the blood vessels so that the heart can pump more easily to supply blood to the rest of the body, thus reducing blood pressure, and aerobic exercise is effective in helping to maintain bone strength.

Stress-busters

Regular exercise can reduce stress dramatically. During periods of high stress, those who reported exercising less frequently had 37 per cent more physical symptoms than their counterparts who exercised more often. In addition, highly stressed people who get less exercise report 21 per cent more anxiety than those who exercise more frequently. Exercise works by using up the adrenaline that is created by stress and stressful situations. It also creates endorphins, the feel-good hormones that improve mood, motivation and even tolerance to pain and other stimuli.

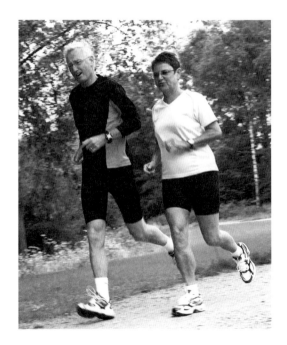

Disease Resistance

Exercise increases health on many levels, and one side-effect is an improved resistance to disease. A study has also shown that physical activity may play a role in deterring cancer, particularly colonic cancer, probably by reducing the amount of time that potential cancer-causing agents take to move through the intestinal system.

Detoxification

Our bodies are designed to cope with a certain number of toxins – those naturally occurring in our foods, for example. Toxins are neutralized, transformed or eliminated by our bodies. The liver helps to transform toxic substances into harmless ones, the intestines break down protein, carbohydrates and fats, while the kidneys filter waste from the bloodstream. We also eliminate toxins through our skin, when we sweat, and our lymphatic system clears debris from our blood. The immune system is also involved – fighting off bacteria and other invaders.

Many therapies initiate a process of detoxification, which means that toxins are forced out of the body, through the use of natural remedies, such as oils, herbs, nutrients and even specific foods. Hydrotherapy and massage can also encourage detoxification. When this happens, you may suffer from symptoms such as headaches, dizziness, bad skin, rashes, diarrhoea, nausea and discharge. These symptoms clear to leave a state of enhanced mental and physical health.

Fasting

Fasting forms a part of naturopathy and a variety of other natural therapies. It serves several purposes; principally it gives the digestive system a rest, detoxifies the system and stimulates the metabolism to get the body up and running so that healing and renewal take place. Naturopaths recommend that most of us should undertake to fast one day a month, even when perfectly healthy.

Diagnosis

Natural practitioners believe that there is something more afoot than simply a physical diagnosis of disease. Indeed, the many elements of health – the mind, body and spirit – are taken into consideration when treating people suffering from virtually any health condition, at any level.

Diagnosis Techniques

Many therapists use a variety of diagnostic techniques alongside the information the patient provides. For example, an Oriental (Chinese, for example) therapist will use personal touch and observation, including:

- ✅ **Pulse-taking (there is more than one pulse in Chinese medicine)**
- ✅ **Abdominal touch**
- ✅ **Posture, movement and skin texture diagnosis**
- ✅ **Tongue diagnosis**
- ✅ **Possible urine analysis**

Other therapists may use some of these techniques:

- ✅ **Radionics:** Using instruments to measure different aspects of your energy state from a 'witness' – a hair clipping or drop of blood – to provide a diagnosis of overall health.

- ✅ **Aura reading:** Many healers appear to be able to read people's auras or energy fields by clairvoyance, touch, or an in-built instinct. Most healers effectively scan the energy field with their hands, sensing areas of heat, cold, pain or tingling which indicate problems. Some therapists actually see and interpret the colours of the aura, and can pick up the effects of past traumas and potential future problems.

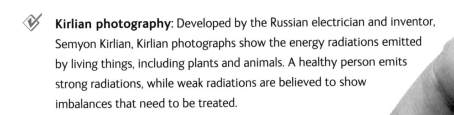

- **Kirlian photography:** Developed by the Russian electrician and inventor, Semyon Kirlian, Kirlian photographs show the energy radiations emitted by living things, including plants and animals. A healthy person emits strong radiations, while weak radiations are believed to show imbalances that need to be treated.

- **Dowsing:** A pendulum is held over the body's energy centres or chakras to indicate strengths and weaknesses in the energy system. It may also be used to give yes/no answers (by swinging clockwise or anti-clockwise) to specific questions about the person's health status and requirements.

- **Iridology:** The iris of the eye represents a map of the glands, organs, and systems of the whole human body. Problems show up on the iris as spots, flecks, white or dark streaks and texture and colour indicate the person's general state of health.

- **Hair analysis:** Chemical analysis of hair is often used to reveal nutritional deficiencies in the body, particularly of minerals.

The Consultation

The consultation is the most important part of any natural therapy session. This is the first session with a therapist, and the one in which the most information is exchanged. The first session usually lasts longer than any subsequent sessions because your therapist will aim to find out all about you as well as your problem before any diagnosis can be made.

Consultation Questions

You can expect your therapist to ask you all about your physical condition, including past and present illnesses, any medication you are taking, any symptoms and interesting aspects to them (sharp pains, or whether they come on in the morning). They will also ask about your diet, including cravings, appetite, any weight problems, alcohol intake, sleeping and exercise patterns.

Importantly, they will also consider your emotional state – are things making you unhappy? Have you recently moved, split up with a partner, lost someone important, failed an important exam? There may also be questions about any other treatment you may be undergoing, either conventional or complementary, and what you hope to get from treatment.

Individual Needs

With this information, the therapist can go ahead and make a diagnosis, which forms the next part of the consultation. After the consultation, treatment can be undertaken, based on your individual needs. The consultation is one aspect of natural medicine that sets it apart from the conventional approach. Sometimes hours are spent ensuring that the therapist has all the information he or she needs to make an informed diagnosis, and

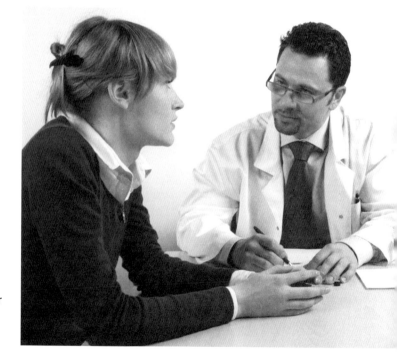

literally get to the bottom of your health problems. The consultation presents a picture of potential causes of the condition, and also provides the therapist with information in order to suggest lifestyle changes.

Radionics

Radionics is based on the belief that the vital energy, or life force, of humans can become blocked, stagnant and thrown into a state of disharmony by infection, stress, pollution, injury, disease, psychological states, malnutrition and poor hygiene.

Practitioners believe that radionics open up the channels of energy so that it flows freely, allowing the body to heal, and reversing the cause of the illness. They claim that every person's energy patterns or rhythms are as unique to them as their fingerprints, and every part of their body, down to cellular level, reflects these vibrations. When illness or disease causes these rhythms to become unbalanced or interrupted, the energy pattern is altered. This altered pattern can be read from any part of the body and treated by sending messages (in a kind of numerical form, with the use of a machine) to the body in order that it may heal itself through a restored flow of energy.

How Radionics Works

A 'witness' – a lock of hair, a drop of blood or a fingernail clipping from the patient – is given to the therapist, who places it in a 'black box' containing various magnets and resistors which will pick up its energy rhythms. Dials on the box are operated until the practitioner senses a resistance, which means that the machine has captured the same energy patterns or rhythm as the witness.

From there, treatment involves sending coded messages back to the patient, through the box, correcting imbalances discovered through the initial analysis. Effectively, the healing energies are transmitted to the patient through the practitioner and the black box. The most remarkable part of the therapy is that there is no need for the patient to be anywhere near the machine for healing to take place. The effects have been felt by patients several thousand miles away. Some radionic practitioners also suggest colour, music, herbs, homeopathy and osteopathy to correct imbalances.

Kinesiology

Kinesiology is a combination of Western technology and the Oriental principles of energy flow. Each of the major organs and systems of the body is fuelled by an invisible channel of energy called a meridian. These channels work together to form a network of energy that powers the mind, all the major functions, organs and muscles of the body.

How Kinesiology Works

When we are healthy, energy flows freely through the channels, but blocked energy can lead to weakness in the corresponding organ and will register in the muscle that relates to that organ. For example, the quadriceps in the front of the thigh are linked by energy to the small intestine and the hamstrings are similarly linked to the large intestine. If you were sensitive to wheat and you ate a piece of bread, the intolerance would register first in the intestines and then in the corresponding muscles in your legs. A kinesiologist would test the strength of the relevant muscle and from there work backwards to find the cause of the problem. This system works for physical, mental and emotional problems.

Kirlian Photography

Kirlian photography was developed in 1939 by the Russian electrician, Semyon Kirlian, and his wife, Valentina. The technique is a way of photographing the quality of the energy of a person or object. It is based on the belief that we are electrical beings and that human electrical energy can be photographed and analyzed. The feet and hands are the parts most commonly photographed.

How Kirlian Photography Works

The participant places a hand or a foot on a machine with photographic plates that emits a high-frequency electrical signal. The image produced indicates the quality of your energy by showing your capacity to resonate with the frequency that is emitted through the plate. The image varies depending on how you feel. The therapist looks at the splines, and at the continuity of the outline of the image, for information about the quality of your energy.

Iridology

According to iridologists, the iris of the eye represents a kind of map of the human glands, organs, and systems of the whole human body. Problems show up on the iris as spots, flecks, and white or dark streaks. Texture and colour indicate the person's general state of health. Some iridologists claim tendencies towards inherited disease and possible future problems are also found and some even address emotional and spiritual health problems this way.

How Iridology Works

Iridology was developed in the nineteenth century by the Hungarian Dr Ignatiz von Peckzely who, as a boy, noticed changes in the eye of an owl with a broken leg. He published his theories in 1881 and soon after, a Swedish doctor, Nils Lilinquist, added his own observations. But iridology did not become widely popular until Dr Bernard Jensen pioneered the use of iridology in the US, eventually, in 1950, publishing a chart that he said showed the location of every gland and organ reflected in each eye.

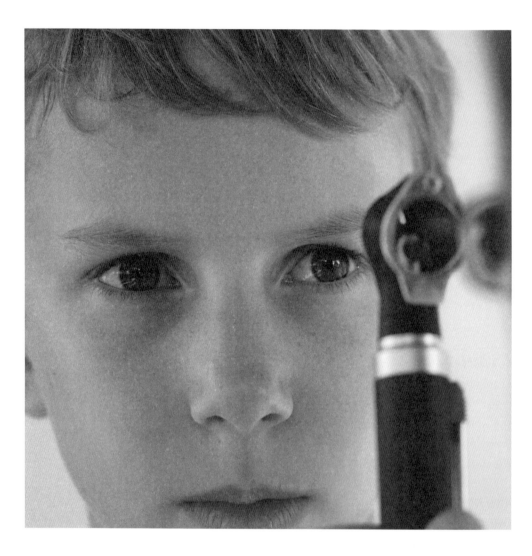

The left eye, he said, corresponds with the left-hand side of the body, the right with the right-hand side. Generally speaking the upper organs (e.g. the brain) are at the top of the iris and the lower ones (e.g. the kidneys) at the bottom. The bodily systems – digestion, blood and lymph, glands and organs, muscles, skeleton and skin – appear in six rings around the pupil.

Iridology Examination

Some practitioners examine the iris with a torch and magnifying glass. Others take colour photographs or transparencies (slides) that are magnified and read. Iridology, or iris diagnosis as it is also known, is widely used by many natural therapists to aid assessment, particularly in the US, Germany and Australia.

Behavioural Therapy

Behavioural therapy, which was introduced at the turn of the twentieth century, is based on learning theories. It aims to predict and control behaviour using scientific means. It concentrates on observing and analysing behaviour and cognitive functioning, diagnosing unproductive habits and ways of dealing with life, and instituting changes in order to change and improve the outcome. Therapists discuss methods and expectations with patients, and the client agrees to participate at a negotiated level. Measures to monitor effectiveness are then established.

Behavioural Therapy Techniques

- **Counter–conditioning**: This involves replacing an undesirable response to a stimulus with a new one.

- **Role playing**: The therapist demonstrates more effective behaviours in a session, which the patients can then apply in real life.

- **Aversion conditioning**: This involves pairing a stimulus that is attractive to the patient but would lead to undesirable results, with an unpleasant event or thought in order to break the pattern.

- **Desensitization**: This involves relaxing the patient and then exposing them gradually and gently to anxiety-provoking situations.

Mental and Emotional Health

In natural medicine, emotional health is considered to be as important as physical health, and is one of the key elements of well-being. Illness is more than just a series of physical symptoms. There is a great deal more involved in ill-health than what is going on in the body.

The Mind-Body Relationship

As adults, we can often sense when we are becoming ill and tend to become irritable, emotional or tearful. We will also succumb to illness more readily during periods of stress, or following a trauma, such as a bereavement or a divorce. The mind-body relationship is not the paragon of alternative medicine alone; there are literally hundreds of scientific studies that show how closely the two are linked.

Health in Balance

When there is an emotional imbalance, physical health can be affected. Similarly, physical health can impact on emotional health. These factors are inextricably intertwined and we need to learn to recognize changes in our emotional health in order to see the whole picture.

Psychotherapy

The mind and emotions are regarded as an integral and vitally important part of total health. All complementary therapies promote the idea of the body as a whole, and that treating it holistically will result in overall health and wellbeing. Psychological influences, such as stress, worry, anxiety and depression can have an enormous impact on health.

Psychotherapies aim to address the parts of the body that some Western medicine has yet to reach successfully. There are a number of types of psychotherapies (properly known as psychological therapies), including behavioural, analytical, humanistic, integrative and even counselling.

Psychotherapy in Practice

Many therapies adopt a form of psychotherapy in their consultation and in further sessions, as a part of treatment. For example, naturopaths approach mental health from the perspective of removing destructive emotions. They are not equipped to deal with serious mental illness such as schizophrenia, but can pinpoint and eliminate the origins of psychosomatic illnesses, mostly through counselling and the use of relaxation techniques.

Counselling

Counselling is a form of treatment for the mind – a form of psychotherapy – and it is not aimed specifically at people who are ill, but at healthy people who wish to deal with a crisis, or improve their lives or relationships. It is, however, often used for relatives of and terminally ill patients, to help them cope with impending death.

Stress Counselling

The link between the mind and body has been long established on scientific grounds, and a physical illness can give rise to psychological symptoms, while an emotional problem can affect overall health. The clearest example of this is stress, which affects both mind and body. Counselling can help people understand the link between various problems and help them learn how to manage them. One of the roles of a natural therapist is to act as a counsellor, encouraging people to express buried emotions and concerns that might be affecting health on all levels. This is one reason why natural medicine is so effective – it addresses the emotional factors with exactly the same emphasis as it does the physical problems.

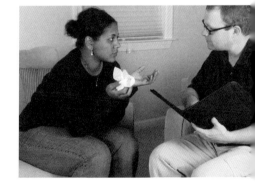

Traditional Therapies

While some naturopathic treatments and diagnostic techniques have developed only in the past century – or even more recently – others have much older roots. Belief in the body's vital force and channels of energy, and the holistic healing associated with it, are ancient eastern traditions.

Traditional Chinese Medicine

Traditional Chinese Medicine (TCM) is a holistic system of medicine that embraces a wide range of therapies, including herbalism, acupuncture, acupressure, diet, massage, exercise (including Qi Gong) and lifestyle factors. It can be enormously helpful for people suffering from chronic and acute health conditions, and for preventative health care.

Applications of TCM

Many conditions can be cured completely with appropriate treatment suggested by a registered TCM practitioner, including asthma, skin diseases, menstrual problems, neurological disorders, allergies, arthritis, depression, digestive disturbances (including colic) and migraine (including abdominal migraine, common in children), colds, coughs, flu, sore throats, period pains (common in young girls), nausea and vomiting, nasal blockages, insomnia, constipation, aches and pains (including growing pains) and earaches.

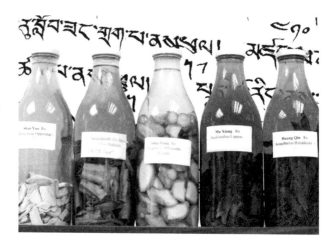

Acupuncture

Acupuncture works by balancing the body's energy to encourage it to heal itself. It can be used to treat a wide range of conditions, including disorders for which conventional medicine has not been able to find a cure or even a cause.

Acupuncture is a medical technique practised in Traditional Chinese Medicine (TCM) and consists of inserting hair-thin needles into the skin at specific points, called acupuncture points or acupoints. It has been used for more than 4,000 years and is used not only for relieving pain but also for curing disease and improving overall health.

The Major Meridians

Chinese medical practitioners believe that a vital force, called *chi*, flows through our body in channels, or meridians. When this vital force, or energy, becomes blocked or stagnant, disease and disharmony result. Acupuncture works by stimulating or relaxing points along the meridians to unblock energy and encourage its flow. Twelve major meridians are identified in acupuncture, although practising acupuncturists make use of 59 major and minor meridians and up to 1,000 acupuncture points along the channels.

What to Expect

The first consultation will last for up to 90 minutes, and your therapist will take great trouble to make an accurate diagnosis, since the success of the treatment depends upon it. He will ask you questions about your health, lifestyle, medical history, symptoms, sleep patterns, sensations of hot and cold, any dizziness, eating habits, bowel movements, emotional problems, relationships and many other factors. He will also note various elements of your appearance, and take pulse readings from each wrist. There are six basic Chinese pulses, three on each wrist. He will then decide on a course of treatment to restore your energy and ensure that you experience optimum health.

The needles will be inserted into the skin and manipulated to calm or stimulate a specific point. He will use up to eight needles, which will either be left in for about 30 minutes, or removed very quickly. Your acupuncturist may also suggest some Chinese herbal treatment, or dietary or lifestyle changes, to go alongside the treatment.

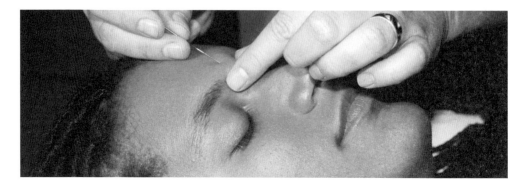

Ayurveda

Ayurveda is the traditional system of healing practised in India and Sri Lanka. Like Traditional Chinese Medicine, Ayurveda is a complete system, with a variety of different components aimed at improving emotional, physical and mental health.

Ayurveda is a Sanskrit word derived from two roots, *ayu* and *vid*, meaning 'life' and 'knowledge'. Ayus, or daily life cycles, represents a combination of the body, the senses organs, the mind and the soul. This science of life embraces both preventative measures and therapeutic procedures, enabling us to improve general health and to become aware of our natural needs and how to satisfy them.

Branches of Ayurveda

Ayurveda is comprised of many different branches, in order to consider all aspects of health and healing. For example, Ayurvedic medicine is only one spoke on the Ayurvedic wheel, and to benefit fully from Ayurveda it is helpful to consider the other elements, including astronomy, meditation, yoga, colour therapy, massage, sound and music therapy, a form of aromatherapy, breathing exercises, and much more.

A Programme for Life

While the approach is vastly different from conventional Western medicine in some ways, it can be considered a programme for living that addresses every part of human life, and puts it into the context of our environment, and even the universe. That is not to say that every element of Ayurveda is essential for health and wellbeing, but by following a simple Ayurvedic approach, we can develop ways of keeping ourselves balanced in times of increasing stress, pressure and worry. Most importantly, however, we can adopt a lifestyle that works to create harmony, preventing illness and encouraging our bodies to heal much more quickly when we do become ill.

Changing Energies

In Ayurveda, it is believed that everything within the universe, including people, is composed of energy, or *prana*. It is because we are made up of constantly changing energy that our bodies, our emotions and our physical environment change in ways that can be both positive and negative. Ayurveda teaches how to encourage the balance of these energies, which means that we are at ease within our bodies and the world around us. Energy controls the functions of every cell, thought, emotion and action, and so all aspects of our lives – including our health, our sleeping patterns, our happiness and well-being, and even our success – can be affected by getting the balance right.

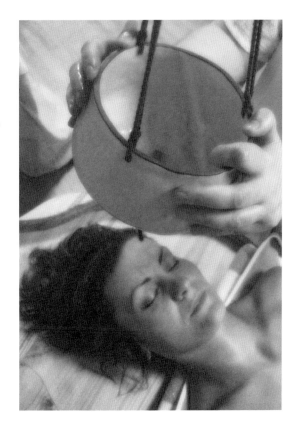

Manipulative Therapies

Manipulative therapies are natural therapies that rely on physical manipulation of the body to create a therapeutic effect. The best-known examples are osteopathy, chiropractic, massage and reflexology. Some of these therapies involve manipulating the whole body, while others focus on smaller parts of the body, such as the hands and feet. Each of these disciplines has its own theory as to how treatment works, but in all, the healing power of touch is relevant to the benefits.

Massage

The therapeutic effects of massage are well-documented, and although sceptics insist that any health benefits derived from treatment are the result of an improved sense of wellbeing, rather than any biological response by the body, there is no doubt that massage works on many levels to improve overall health.

Benefits of Massage

Massage is one of the oldest, simplest forms of therapy and is a system of stroking, pressing and kneading different areas of the body to relieve pain, relax, stimulate and tone the body. Massage does much more than make you feel good, it also works on the soft tissues (the muscles, tendons and ligaments) to improve muscle tone. Although it largely affects those muscles just under the skin, it is believed that it also reaches the deeper layers of muscles and possibly even the organs themselves.

Effects on Blood Flow

Massage is known to increase the circulation of blood and the flow of lymph. The direct mechanical effect of rhythmically applied manual pressure and movement used in massage can dramatically increase the rate of blood flow. Also, the stimulation of nerve receptors causes the blood vessels (by relaxation) to dilate, which also encourages blood flow.

For the whole body to be healthy, the individual cells must be healthy. These cells are dependent on an abundant supply of blood and lymph because these fluids supply nutrients and oxygen and carry away wastes and toxins. It causes changes in the blood. The oxygen capacity of the blood can increase 10–15 per cent after massage.

Muscular Benefits

Massage can help loosen contracted, shortened muscles and can stimulate weak, flaccid muscles. This muscle balancing can help posture and promote more efficient movement. Massage does not directly increase muscle strength, but it can speed recovery from the fatigue that occurs after exercise. Massage also provides a gentle stretching action to both the muscles and connective tissues that surround and support the muscles and many other parts of the body, which helps keep these tissues elastic.

Stimulation

It increases the body's secretions and excretions. There is a proven increase in the production of gastric juices, saliva and urine. There is also increased excretion of nitrogen, inorganic phosphorus and sodium chloride (salt), suggesting that the metabolic rate (the utilization of absorbed material by the body's cells) increases.

Massage balances the nervous system by soothing or stimulating it, depending on what you need at the time of the massage. Massage directly improves the function of the sebaceous (oil) and sweat glands, which keep the skin lubricated, clean and cooled. Tough, inflexible skin can become softer and more supple. By indirectly or directly stimulating the nerves that supply internal organs, blood vessels of the organs dilate and allow greater blood supply to reach them.

Shiatsu

Shiatsu is a Japanese form of body work. It was developed from different disciplines of Oriental medicine, including acupuncture, herbalism, diet and exercise. Shiatsu, like many forms of massage, works to relax and invigorate the body. Shiatsu also makes use of the energy of the body and originated as a holistic therapy for the treatment of mind, body and spirit. When used correctly it remains a holistic therapy, taking into consideration the mind, body and spirit. It is as useful for emotional pain as it is for physical problems.

How Shiatsu Works

The word shiatsu can be broken down into *shi*, which means 'finger' and *atsu*, which means 'pressure'. In reality shiatsu may be thumb, finger, elbow or even knee pressure. The quality of the pressure is the main feature that differentiates shiatsu from other forms of massage. To work with the body's energy the pressure must reach through the superficial layers of the body to its centre. Sometimes this feels deeply relaxing and sometimes this can be quite sharp.

Shiatsu is given on a Japanese mattress which means the giver and the receiver are at floor level. The receiver remains clothed which helps the practitioner contact the body's energy rather than the skin. Shiatsu involves the giver leaning on the receiver and moving along the meridians. Shiatsu differs from an oil massage as there are moments of stillness in the movement for the giver to contact the energy.

Benefits of Shiatsu

Shiatsu at the hands of a qualified therapist is perfectly safe for everyone and particularly beneficial for pregnant women. Some therapists also specialise in the treatment of small children and the elderly. Shiatsu is not suitable, however, for people with cancer of the blood or lymphatic systems. Done correctly, shiatsu:

 Relaxes

 Restores and balances energy

Eases tension and stiffness

 Improves breathing

 Improves circulation

 Heals the body and mind

Enhances well-being

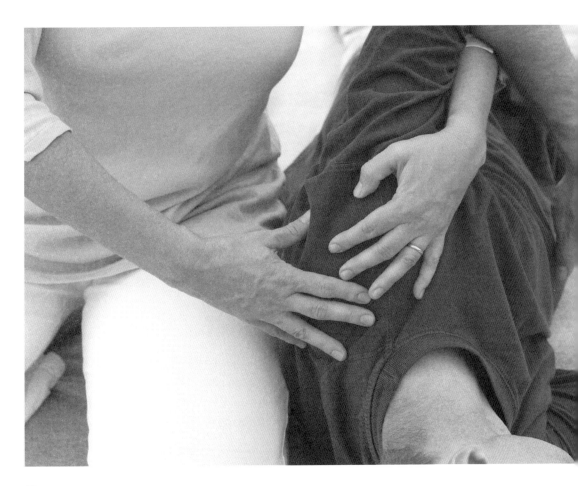

Acupressure

Acupressure is one of the most ancient healing traditions, perhaps predating acupuncture itself. The Chinese discovered that pressure on specific points of the body could relieve common health problems. Acupressure is based on the same concept of meridians and acupoints in acupuncture but fingertip pressure is applied rather than needles. The aim is to balance the flow of energy within the meridians to ensure that all organs and body systems are functioning well. In this way disease is prevented or cured.

How Acupressure Works

Acupressure is similar to Shiatsu in that it involves the use of finger pressure on acupuncture points to stimulate the smooth flow of *chi* (energy) through the channels of the body. Unlike shiatsu, acupressure involves mostly thumb and fingertip pressure, although it can also incorporate massage along the meridians. Pressure is used evenly and applied in the direction of the flow of the meridians. Pressure may also be applied using small wooden sticks with rounded ends for single points or rollers for covering several points simultaneously.

Acupressure is used to relieve a number of common ailments including headaches, back pain, fatigue, constipation, and is particularly useful for stress-related disorders such as digestive problems, mood swings, insomnia and even asthma. It can be self-administered, although knowledge of acupoints and meridians is essential to ensure that the proper points are being treated.

Chiropractic

The word chiropractic comes from the Greek *cheir* which means 'hand' and *praktikos* meaning 'done by'. Manipulation of the body has been practised for thousands of years by ancient cultures such as the Greeks, the Egyptians and the Chinese. Even Hippocrates, the father of medicine, suggested that knowledge of the spine was necessary for understanding and treating disease.

Spinal Problems

Our spinal cord is enclosed by 24 movable vertebrae. Between each vertebra various nerves branch out to every part of the body. If a vertebra is slightly displaced, it can interfere with the spinal cord and the nerves. Chiropractors believe that this slight misalignment may cause problems across the whole body, affecting the way our bodies function.

How Chiropractic Works

Chiropractors work to eliminate imbalances causing medical problems by manipulating the spine with their hands to realign the vertebrae. Pain is a message from the body indicating distress or dysfunction on some level. If it is caught early enough, this dysfunction can be treated with chiropractic adjustments that may help the body to heal itself. When pain is ignored, the immune system and parts of the body that control pain become overwhelmed and unable to cope and our body begins to descend into disease and ill-health.

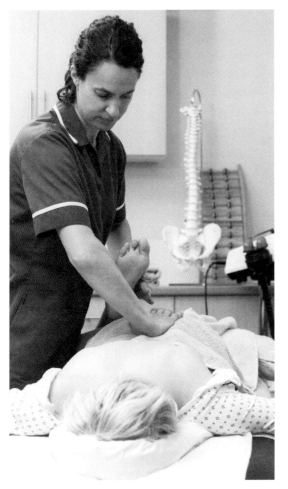

Treatment may involve soft tissue work and then manipulation. They can sometimes feel uncomfortable, but the types of treatment and the amount of pressure used are tailored to the individual. Often very little force is necessary. All treatment is undertaken according to a patient's specific symptoms, level of health, age and build.

Benefits of Chiropractic Treatment

Chiropractors treat any kind of pain or condition relating to the muscles and skeleton and the associated nervous system. Treatable conditions include neuritis, sciatica, neuralgia, muscular pains, migraines, headaches, stress and its related disorders (fatigue, insomnia, anxiety and digestive disorders), some asthma conditions, bad posture, sprained muscles and ligaments, accident-related injuries, rheumatism and arthritis.

Osteopathy

Osteopathy, like chiropractic, is a manipulative therapy based on the belief that the skeleton and organ systems are dependent upon one another, and therefore body functions will only work effectively if body structure is properly aligned. Misalignment of the spine and skeleton can cause organs to dysfunction and impairs the circulation of blood and lymph.

The Philosophy of Osteopathy

Most osteopaths will work on posture, joints and muscles, not just to correct structural problems, but because structural integrity also affects internal organs and tissue. Structural disorders can also be affected by unhealthy emotional problems, especially in the case of recurring conditions. Osteopaths work on the soft tissue of the body using a specific type of manipulation.

Osteopaths believe that we function as a complete working system – our body structure, organs, systems, mind and emotions are all interrelated and mutually interdependent. Consequently, problems that affect the structural body upset the balance of the body generally. Similarly, internal problems can reveal themselves in the body's structure as it adapts to accommodate pain, discomfort or disease. By manipulating the body structure, osteopaths aim to restore health and balance in the whole person, not just at the site of pain.

Muscular Relief

Much of osteopathic practice focuses on easing muscular tension, which does more than simply alleviate pain and stiffness. The osteopathic belief that a relaxed muscle is a well-functioning muscle is based on the physiological fact that muscles use up an enormous amount of the body's energy when they contract. Stress, either mental or physical, can cause muscles to contract, wasting energy and making the muscles less elastic so that they are more prone to damage.

Tense muscles can also impede the circulation of blood and lymph which flow through them. By relaxing tight muscles these important fluids can flow freely, allowing blood to carry nutrients and oxygen to where they are needed and enabling waste-carrying lymph to drain them away. The ribs and diaphragm are also surrounded by muscles. Work in this area can improve existing respiratory conditions such as asthma and chronic bronchitis.

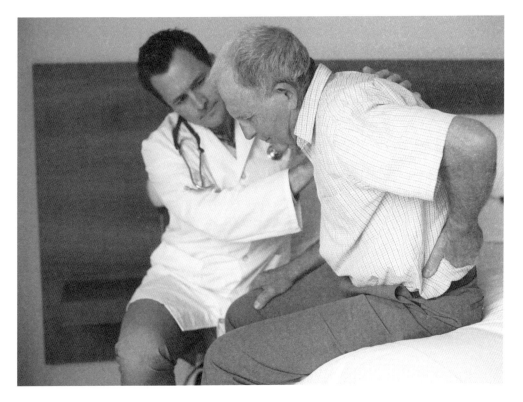

Cranial Osteopathy

Cranial osteopathy was developed in the 1930s by American osteopath, William Garner Sutherland. His training taught him that the bones of the skull, which are separate at birth, grew together into a fixed structure and so could not move. He also noticed, however, that the bones of the skull retained some potential for movement even into adulthood. If they could move, they could also be susceptible to dysfunction.

Sutherland discovered that the fluid around the spinal cord and brain had detectable rhythms, which he called 'the breath of life', as the rhythms appeared to be influenced by the rate and depth of breathing. By gently manipulating the skull he found he could alter the rhythm of this fluid flow and suggested that it might stimulate the body's self-healing ability and help to heal conditions which appeared unrelated to the cranium.

Cranial Rhythm

The human skull is made up of some 26 bones which are not fixed but can move slightly. Inside the skull the brain is surrounded by cerebrospinal fluid. The fluid is secreted in the brain and from there flows out of the skull and down the spine, enveloping the spinal cord and the base of the spinal nerves. Practitioners believe that cerebrospinal fluid is pumped through the spinal canal by means of a pulsation, which has its own rhythm, unrelated to the heartbeat or the breathing mechanism. When the bones of the skull move normally the cranial rhythm remains balanced, but any disturbance to the cranial bones can disturb the normal motion of the bones and consequently alter the cranial rhythm. This affects the functioning of other parts of the body.

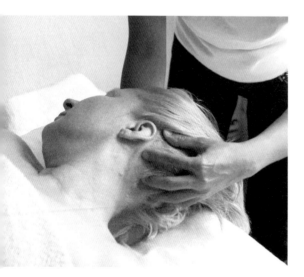

How Cranial Osteopathy Works

A trained osteopath can feel the rhythm of the cranial pulse anywhere in the body, but principally at the skull and the sacrum. By holding and exerting very gentle pressure on the skull the practitioner can feel the rhythm of the cranial pulse and detect irregularities. The technical approach used involves extremely gentle, but specifically applied adjustments to the movement of body tissues. Cranial osteopathy is both gentle and non-invasive, making it a very safe method of diagnosis and treatment for even newborn babies.

There are many conditions that have been successfully treated by cranial osteopathy, including asthma, co-ordination difficulties, dental problems, digestive problems, dyslexia, glue ear, hyperactivity, colic, sleeping problems, migraines and headaches, digestive disorders, speech problems and also scoliosis (abnormal curvature of the spine).

Rolfing

Rolfing is named after its founder, Dr Ida Rolf (1896–1979), an American biochemist. Rolfing is intended to integrate manipulative forms of treatment with bioenergetics (the study of energy in living things). When our bodies are well-aligned, gravity can flow through us, allowing ease of movement. A poor alignment is pulled down by gravity and struggles to keep balance, compensating and making changes until the entire structure is weakened.

Benefits of Rolfing

Rolfing realigns body structure and restores balance. It relies mainly on deep massage of the muscles and connective tissues, to return the body to a state of balance. When the body is balanced, the mind, nervous system and all the organs and tissues to which it relates can function more efficiently. The body's innate healing system can therefore work at optimum level.

Movement and psychology have become part of training, so both emotional and physical problems can be dealt with. Rolfing is best used for ailments affecting the musculoskeletal system (caused by mechanical stress), poor posture and breathing difficulties.

Reflexology

Reflexology involves stimulating, massaging and applying pressure to points on the hands and feet which correspond to various systems and organs throughout the body in order to stimulate the body's own healing system. These points are called reflex points, and each point corresponds to a different body part or function.

Benefits of Reflexology

Reflexologists believe that applying pressure to these reflex points can improve the health of the body and mind. Depending on the points chosen, reflexology can be used to ease tension, reduce inflammation, relieve congestion, improve circulation and eliminate toxins from the body. Like many other complementary therapists, reflexologists do not claim to cure anything, rather they aim to stimulate the body to heal itself. They do this by working on the physical body to stimulate the healing at the physical, mental and emotional levels.

Pressure applied to nerve endings can influence all the body systems, including the circulation and lymphatic systems. Improvements in circulation and the lymphatic system result in improved body functioning because nutrients and oxygen are transported more efficiently around the body and toxins are eliminated with greater ease. Energy pathways are opened up so that the body is able to work more effectively, and harmony or 'homeostasis' is restored.

Reflex Zones

Reflexologists believe that the body is divided into 10 vertical zones or channels, five on the left and five on the right. Each zone runs from the head right down to the reflex areas on the hands and feet, and from the front through to the back of the body. All the body parts within any one zone are linked by nerve pathways and are mirrored in the corresponding reflex zone on the hands and feet. By applying pressure to a reflex point or area, the therapist can stimulate or rebalance the energy in the related zone.

Each zone is a channel for energy, and stimulating or working any zone in the foot by applying pressure with the thumbs and fingers affects the entire zone throughout the body. For example, working a zone on the foot along which the kidneys lie will release vital energy that may be blocked somewhere else in that zone, such as in the eyes. Working the kidney reflex area on the foot will therefore revitalize and balance the entire zone and improve functioning of the organ.

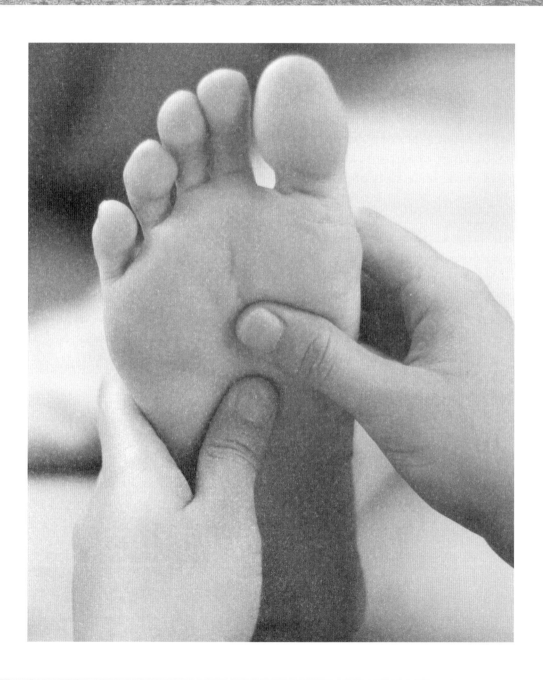

Other Therapies

While massage and other manipulative therapies might be the best-known naturopathic practices, there are many other therapies available that can treat a range of ailments and imbalances. Although often focused on specific parts of the body, they are still based on the principles of holistic healing.

Sound Therapy

Sound therapy is an ancient method of healing. The theory is that as everything in the Universe is in a constant state of vibration, including the human body, even the smallest change in frequency can affect the internal organs. Modern sound therapists consider that there is a natural resonance or 'note' for each part of the body, and for each individual. They direct specific sound waves to specific areas to affect the frequency at which that part is vibrating. In this way, health is restored and balanced.

How Sound Therapy Works

Sound therapy may use machines that transmit healing vibrations, but more usually it involves direct application of the voice, music or a combination of sounds. Specifically directed sounds can be used in the treatment of a variety of disorders, and have been very effective in the past with disabled children and adults.

Auricular therapy

Auricular therapy is ear acupuncture. According to auricular therapists there are many benefits. Firstly, it provides quick access to diagnostic information, and you do not have to be treated with needles. Therapists can use very fine, small needles that go in to a depth of only one millimetre, but they can also use light therapy, electrotherapy or very small magnetically charged ball bearings, which press on the relevant points.

Other Advantages

You can have semi-permanent treatment. Small needles can be embedded in the ear or small ball bearings can be taped over the necessary points for up to a week at a time. This way you can press on the point when you feel the need. It is less invasive than body acupuncture and so is better for patients who are anxious about their problem or the treatment, or who are reluctant to undress for treatment. It is an effective form of pain control with an immediate calming effect.

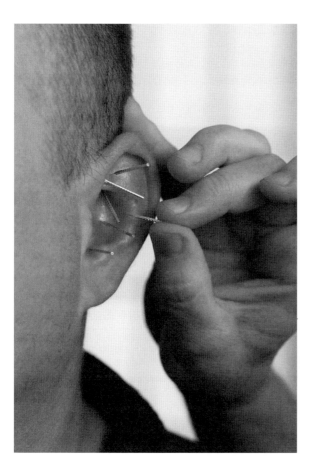

Needling

The ear is believed to mirror the shape of the foetus in the womb: the lobe represents the head, and points relating to the tongue, eyes, tonsils, teeth and ears are all found on the lobe. The rest of the points are positioned on the ear where they would exactly match the organs to which they correspond if a miniature foetus were superimposed over the ear. Opinions vary as to how many points there are on the ear, some say there are 200, others say it is over 300, but each one relates to a specific organ or area of the body. Needling, or otherwise stimulating a point on the ear, affects the corresponding organ or meridian in the same way that stimulating a point on the body would.

Polarity Therapy

Polarity therapy is the science of balancing opposite energies within the body to promote mental, physical and emotional health. It is a combination of Eastern and Western approaches to health. The name 'polarity' was chosen to convey the image of the body as a living magnet, where electromagnetic energy flows between its positive and negative poles.

Principles of Polarity Therapy

According to polarity therapy, disease can go by many names, but ultimately the only cause of disease is blocked energy. Energy can become blocked by internal emotional stresses or by external factors such as poor diet and lack of energy. Once unblocked, free-flowing energy can again restore mind and body to health.

The therapy is based on the belief that the body is governed by the opposite poles of positive and negative, similar to the Chinese philosophy of the opposites of yin and yang. Energy is seen as electromagnetic, so in order for it to flow around the body it must have poles to flow between. The flow of energy is governed by five energy centres in the body, called chakras. Chakras are like energy substations, constantly working to replenish stores of energy and generate it through the whole person.

Techniques

The role of polarity therapy is not simply to unblock the energy, but to help you resolve the problems that created the blockages in the first place. To do this the polarity therapist uses four techniques:

 Bodywork: Using touch on specific parts of the body to balance, remove blocks and improve vitality.

 Awareness skills: Teaching that shock and overwhelming situations can be held in the body's energy, causing blockage; therapists help you work through issues to prevent energy from being affected.

Diets: Prescribed according to your specific type and characteristics; detoxification, to unblock and stimulate energy, is often advised, as is maintaining an acid/alkaline balance.

 Exercise: Stretching postures are a series of yoga-type postures for each chakra that are designed to release stagnant energy.

Reiki

Reiki means 'universal life energy' in Japanese, and it is a form of healing based on tapping into the unseen flow of energy that permeates all living things. It is believed that reiki originally evolved as a branch of Tibetan Buddhism, and that knowledge of its power and use was transmitted from master to disciple.

Reiki in Practice

Treatment by a reiki master is intended to promote physical, emotional and spiritual wellbeing. Clients lie or sit fully clothed while the practitioner's hands are placed on specific parts of the body, starting with the head. Some reiki practitioners do not touch the physical body, but transmit healing into the aura around the body.

Benefits of Reiki

Reiki is aimed at encouraging the healing energies in the body, and involves transmitting the healer's own energy to the sufferer. Most emotional, physical and spiritual conditions will respond to treatment, including many that are considered to be untreatable by the conventional medical profession.

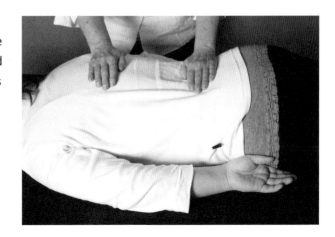

Cymatics

Cymatics was developed in the 1960s by British medical doctor and osteopath Dr Peter Manners. The therapy grew out of early research into electromagnetic energy and the concept that every living thing – person, animal, plant or organism – is surrounded by an energy field that resonates at its own particular frequency.

Principles of Cymatics

Cymatics comes from the Greek word *kyma*, meaning 'a great wave'. Cymatic therapy is a form of sound therapy, based on the principle that every cell in the body – of which there are believed to be 60 million – is controlled by an electromagnetic field that resonates at its own particular sound frequency. When we are well this frequency is constant, but dysfunction or disease upsets the harmony of the body and the area affected generates an increased resonance.

Healing Through Cymatics

The practitioner uses the cymatic machinery to generate a frequency identical to that of healthy cells. His aim is to support what the cell is trying to do naturally, therefore empowering the healing process and restoring the body to health and harmony.

Hydrotherapy

Hydrotherapy, or water therapy, can be used to improve circulation and increase vitality so that the vital force can work more efficiently. It can also be used to ease pain. Hot, cold and alternate hot and cold water are used to achieve specific effects. Hot water is initially stimulating but has a secondary relaxing effect. Cold water is also stimulating with an invigorating and tonic effect. Alternate hot and cold baths or showers stimulate blood and lymph circulation, help to remove congestion and have a tonic effect on body tissues.

Types of Hydrotherapy

Naturopaths use many forms of water therapy, such as cold compresses which are used to boost the elimination of toxins, cold baths, hot baths, saunas, and sitz baths. Sitz baths are hip baths where you sit alternately in hot and cold water. They are believed to be particularly helpful in pelvic disorders such as fibroids, constipation and haemorrhoids. Epsom salts baths are commonly recommended by naturopaths and are valued for the cleansing effect they have on the body.

Internal uses of hydrotherapy such as enemas and colonic irrigation are sometimes used, but their use is a cause of some debate, even among naturopaths.

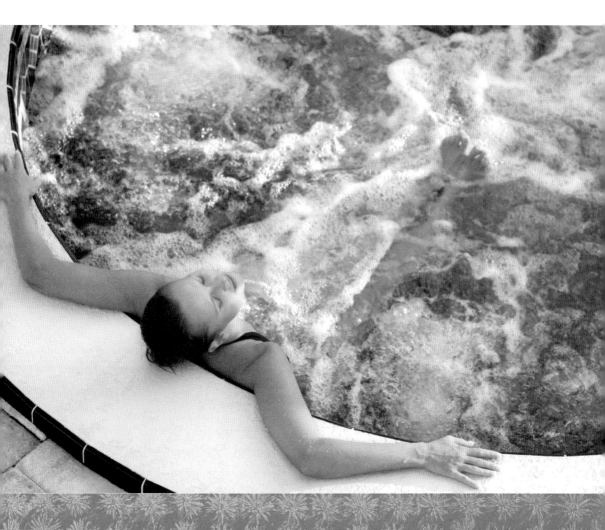

Crystals and Gemstones

For thousands of years crystals have been credited with mystical and healing powers. They were used by ancient astrologers, diviners and priests and have long been revered for their beauty and power. Today, crystals are used for their unique healing powers, and crystal and gem therapy have become popular forms of treatment.

Crystal Therapy

A crystal is defined as a mineral that has a definite atomic structure, with smooth, flat faces arranged in a geometric pattern. Every crystal is believed to be a perfect example of organized matter. Tuning into the perfection of the crystal is believed to bring the individual closer to perfection.

Crystals are believed to exert positive healing energies that can help to rebalance us because they match the energy of the human aura very well. Crystals can generate, store and give off electromagnetic energy. Each crystal has its own particular energy that vibrates at a level that can have specific healing effects on mind, body and spirit.

How Does Crystal Therapy Work?

Like many other therapies, crystals work on an energy level, or a 'vibrational' basis. Everything in our physical environment is comprised of energy; in fact, humans are simply dense bodies of energy. This energy can be depleted or become imbalanced by numerous external and internal influences, from thinking negatively to eating the wrong foods and absorbing radiation from computer screens.

Crystals vibrate with energy that has the potential to alter our energy flow, and they work in a similar way to flower essences. A crystal therapist will adapt their own treatment, depending on your individual requirements. They may place crystals around your chair or couch to surround you with healing energy, or they may give you a crystal to hold. Some therapists will place crystals on the body's seven energy centres, known as chakras.

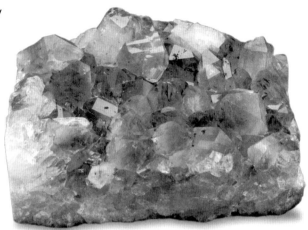

If you have physical pain, the therapist may place a crystal over the site of the pain. Energy from the crystal then passes through the body to the point of pain or imbalance. The crystals can be left in place for a few seconds or for several minutes, it varies enormously depending on the site and intensity of the pain. The choice of the crystal or crystals depends on what the therapist believes to be your own particular needs.

Gem Therapy

Gemstones such as emeralds, garnet and jade vibrate with energy. They are used like other crystals, but are also used to create gem essences. These work in a similar way to flower essences. The stones are immersed in purified water and left in the sunshine, so that the sun's rays transmit the energy from the gem to the water. The same effect is sometimes achieved using a pyramid, pendulum or the energy of a healer. The energized water is then poured into small bottles, which you can use by either holding in your hand for several minutes or by placing a few drops under the tongue. Not all gems are suitable for essences as some, such as turquoise and malachite, contain copper and are poisonous.

More than 200 gem and mineral essences have been created in the belief that they will assist the healing of specific mental and emotional states.

Exercise and Meditation

Most naturopaths recognize the importance of both exercise and relaxation in the process of holistic healing. Therapists use and teach a number of different types of physical and mental relaxation techniques and in some cases induce very deep relaxation.

Relaxation and Breathing

It has been found that relaxation can reduce the heart rate, lower blood pressure, and regulate breathing and metabolic rate. It also reduces adrenaline levels and allows the immune system to function more efficiently. Stress is a normal and necessary part of life, which provides motivation, stimulation and the drive to meet challenges with enthusiasm. The key to controlling it is relaxation.

Relaxing for Healing

True relaxation is a healing process that focuses on relaxing the mind and body. You will learn how to control and resolve the effects of stress rather than suppressing them with short-term measures, such as alcohol or overeating. Relaxation is a skill. Practised correctly, it can both prevent and treat disease, and improve your sense of wellbeing. Once you have learned how to do it, relaxation is a state that you can bring about wherever you are and whatever you are doing.

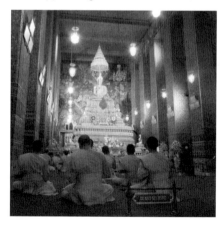

Meditation

The word meditation comes from the Latin *meditori*, meaning 'to reflect on'. Western medicine has been slow to catch on to the benefits of meditation, but research has now shown that it can slow your heart rate, reduce negative emotions and produce a sense of calm. Meditation is a tool to make us aware of the peace within us, a place that the outside world cannot touch or influence.

Yoga

Yoga encourages better breathing and relaxation. Used therapeutically, yoga can help with the following: muscle joint mobility, flexibility, breathing disorders, musculoskeletal pain, nervous system and endocrine disorders, digestive problems, fatigue, insomnia and stress-related conditions.

Body in Harmony

The word yoga means 'unity' or 'oneness' and is derived from the Sanskrit word *yug* which means 'to join'. In spiritual terms it refers to the union of the individual consciousness with the universal consciousness. On a practical level yoga is a means of balancing and harmonizing the body, mind and emotions, and is a tool that allows us to withdraw from the chaos of the world and find a quiet space within. It utilizes the innate life force within the body and teaches how to tap into, harness and direct it skilfully. To achieve this, yoga uses movement, breath, posture, relaxation and meditation in order to establish a healthy, vibrant and balanced approach to living.

Yoga Postures

Yoga exercises are comprised of *asanas*, or postures, that involve stretching, bending, turning and relaxation. Each posture has a specific therapeutic effect. There are six main groups of yoga postures: standing, inverted, twist, back bend, forward bend and side bend.

 Standing: Improves efficiency of the muscular, circulatory, respiratory, digestive, reproductive, endocrine and nervous systems.

 Inverted: Balances endocrine system and metabolism. Enhances thinking power and revitalizes internal organs.

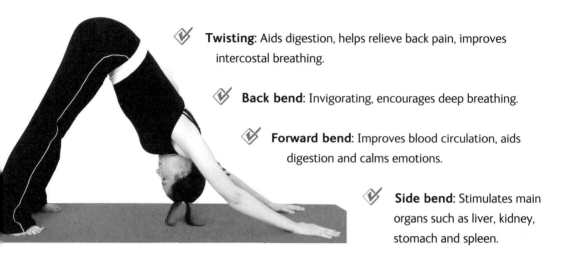

Twisting: Aids digestion, helps relieve back pain, improves intercostal breathing.

Back bend: Invigorating, encourages deep breathing.

Forward bend: Improves blood circulation, aids digestion and calms emotions.

Side bend: Stimulates main organs such as liver, kidney, stomach and spleen.

Alexander Technique

The Alexander Technique is not a therapy as such, but a process of re-education, which aims to teach us to rediscover our natural poise, grace and freedom and use our bodies more efficiently. It is taught in lessons where the practitioner is referred to as a teacher, not a therapist, and the individual participating in the lessons is known as a pupil, not a patient or client.

Principles

The Alexander Technique works on the principle that mind and body form a complex and integrated whole. As a holistic system, the technique is not taught in order to alleviate specific ailments, such as a stiff neck or aching back, but is concerned with addressing the source of such problems. However, it has been found that in the process of restoring harmony to the whole person, specific problems often disappear.

When taught by a qualified teacher, the Alexander Technique is safe for everyone to use. Young children do not usually need it as they have natural poise and balance, but they can be taught it as a preventative technique. Children with physical handicaps, such as polio and scoliosis of the spine, can also benefit from it. The technique is perfectly safe to learn at any stage of pregnancy. Pregnant women may find that it helps them cope with their changing shape and the pressure it puts on their spine. Many women who learnt it during pregnancy believe it enabled them to have an easier labour.

Benefits of the Alexander Technique

The Alexander Technique is not a cure for any condition or illness, although many symptoms appear to improve during practice. To date, there is not much scientific evidence for the benefits of this technique, but students and teachers report an improvement in numerous problems. Stress-related conditions, general fatigue and lethargy, anxiety, breathing disorders, back, neck and joint pain are believed to be improved.

It has also been shown to help in the recovery from illness or injury and is believed to increase self-awareness and improve both personal and professional relationships. Actors, singers and dancers claim it enhances their performance and sports men and women believe it improves their co-ordination and helps them to use their energy more efficiently.

Dance Therapy

Dance therapy uses movement and dance to explore how a patient's emotional disturbance is linked to their bodily experiences. A dance therapist observes and analyzes how you express yourself through the use of your body, assesses your strengths and identifies areas in which you might benefit from therapy. The therapist may also work with you on an individual basis, using movements designed to help you build a stronger sense of your own identity.

Interpreting Movement

Movement can also be used to help resolve issues that may have occurred before you learnt to speak, when movement was your natural means of expression. In group work the therapist notes how members share emotional expression, assesses how the group works together and judges when to intervene. For example, introducing the concept of leading and following may help to draw someone out of their self-preoccupied isolation.

A therapist will have various pieces of equipment such as balls, beanbags and stretch cloths in the room, which can be used by the group to explore particular themes. Members of the group, for example, can pull and release cloths while exploring the theme of trust.

T'ai Chi

T'ai chi or t'ai chi ch'uan means 'supreme ultimate power' and is often referred to as 'meditation in motion'. A Chinese martial art, t'ai chi was founded by a Taoist monk more than 5,000 years ago. Chairman Mao incorporated it into general Chinese health practice in

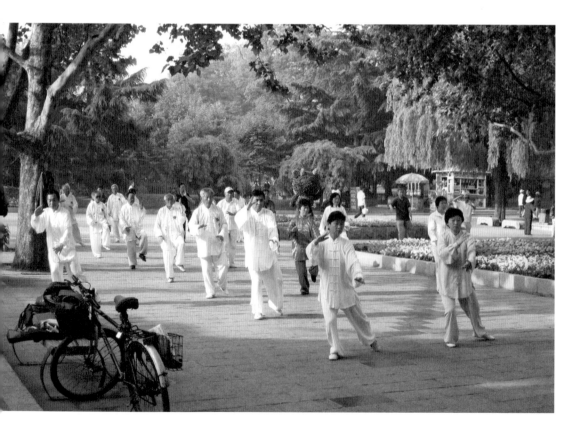

1949 in order to relieve stress and associated disorders. Derived from Confucian, Buddhist and Taoist teachings, this art or therapy is a complete physical and mental discipline, which promotes health and well-being.

Stimulating the Chi

T'ai chi is a series of flowing actions based on the movements of nature. The Chinese theory of *chi*, or energy, is incorporated into this discipline, and this therapy is designed to gently stir or stimulate the flow of *chi* to unblock any points of stagnation or poor circulation, and allow the flow to reach any weakened parts of the body. Illness and disease are believed to be the result of an imbalance of chi in the body.

Traditionally t'ai chi has 128 postures, all of which must be taught and worked through at a specific, slow pace. These postures run together in a flowing movement, which can have a powerful effect on physical and psychological health.

Biofeedback

Biofeedback is a form of technologically supported relaxation therapy that was developed in the US. Patients are taught a series of relaxation exercises similar to autogenic training (a relaxation technique designed to influence the autonomic nervous system, during which you repeat a set of visualisations that induce a state of relaxation), but in biofeedback it is taken one step further and a patient's progress is monitored by machines which assess changes in heart rate, body temperature, muscle tension, skin conductivity and brain waves.

Once training is complete, patients learn how to recognize their body's signals and reach a state of relaxation themselves, which is the basis of the therapy. Biofeedback trains patients to recognize the symptoms of stress, migraines, or whatever illness they suffer from, and then to take the appropriate steps to deal with them. The most common conditions that benefit from biofeedback are stress and anxiety related disorders such as insomnia, digestive troubles, headaches and high blood pressure.

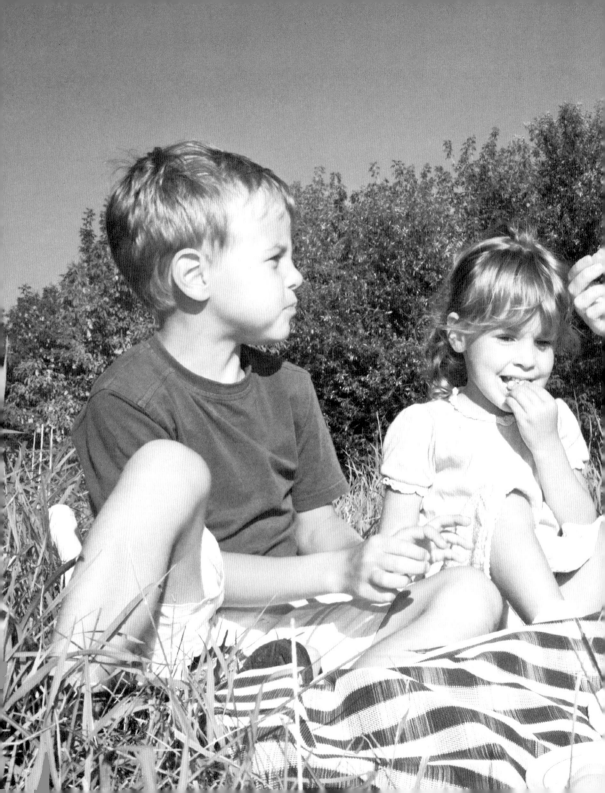

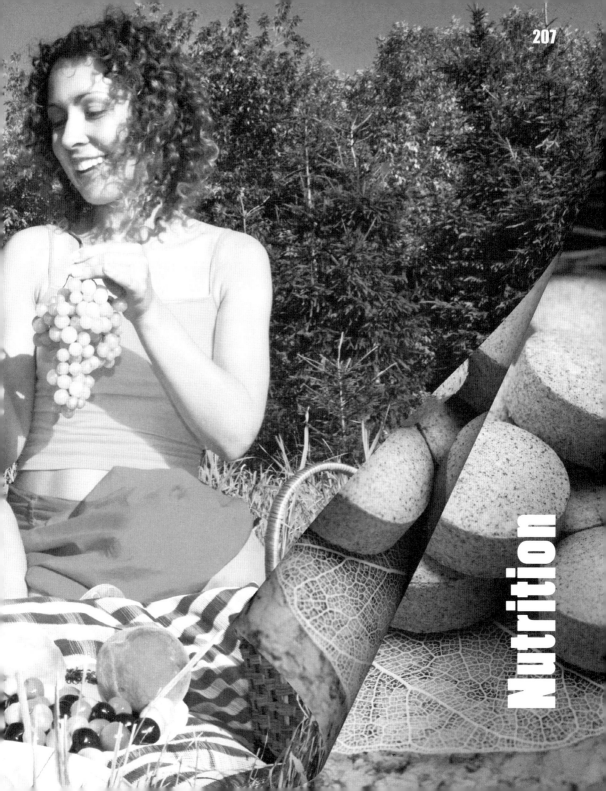

Nutrition

Understanding Nutrition

Our understanding of vitamins, minerals and other micronutrients, compounds and elements – and their role in our bodies – has improved dramatically over the decades. We now know that 'micronutrition' – or the vitamins, minerals and other health-giving components of our food, such as amino acids, fibre, enzymes and lipids – is crucial to life.

Everyday Nutrition

We now know that by manipulating our nutritional intake, we can not only ensure good health and address ailments, but also prevent illness and some of the degenerative effects of ageing. Exciting new discoveries related to the nutrient components of our food mean that more than half of us are now taking supplements in one form or another, convinced that diet itself – bearing in mind the stresses on our body and the polluted world in which we live – is inadequate to supply us with our nutritional needs.

The Development of Naturopathic Nutrition

In the late-nineteenth century naturopaths drew attention to the use of food and its nutritional elements as medicine, a concept that was not new, but which had not been acknowledged as a therapy in its own right until that time. Naturopaths used nutrition and fasting to cleanse the body, and to encourage its ability to heal itself. As knowledge about food, its make-up, and the effects it has on our body became greater with the development of biochemistry, the first nutritional specialists undertook to treat specific ailments and symptoms with the components of food.

Body Biochemistry

By the middle of the twentieth century, scientists had put together a profile of proteins, carbohydrates and fats, as well as vitamins and minerals, which were essential to life and to health. More than 40 nutrients were uncovered, including 13 vitamins. It was discovered that minerals were needed for body functions, and a new understanding of the body and its biochemistry fed the growing interest in the subject.

In the 1960s, doctors began to treat patients with special diets and supplements, prescribed according to individual symptoms, problems and needs. While conventional medical doctors still discussed nutrition in terms of basic food groups, nutritionists were prescribing vitamins in mega-doses. Other elements and compounds were soon identified as necessary to human life, and we are now able to purchase and take substances like amino acids, bee pollen, lipids (such as evening primrose oil and cod-liver oil), seaweeds, acidophilus (healthy bacteria) and dietary enzymes.

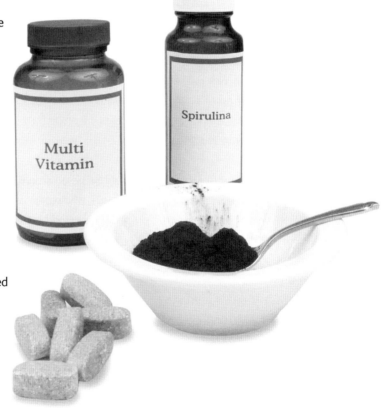

Holistic Nutrition

Nutrition has changed from being a mainly doctor-led dietary therapy, also called clinical nutrition, into a more profound theory of health based on treating the patient as a whole (holistic health), and looking for deficiencies that may be causing illness which are specific to each individual.

Diet

Diet is an essential part of every single natural therapy, as it forms the foundation of our overall health. Everything we eat has the power to enhance or detract from our health. We now know, for example, that 80 per cent of all cancers are linked to diet. So are fertility, heart disease, immune function, mental prowess, weight, the health of our bones and teeth, allergies and, of course, wellbeing.

Healthy Food vs. Junk Food

In the West, we have adopted a diet based around pre-packaged, easy-to-cook or 'instant' convenience foods. Not only are these poor in the essential nutrients required for growth and the functioning of every system in our bodies, but they contain a host of chemicals that put a strain on our bodies and act as anti-nutrients, meaning they actually use up what little nutrition we do get in order to process the 'junk'.

A healthy diet is easy to achieve and should be based around wholefoods in their natural state. In other words, wholegrain breads are far superior to white processed breads and brown rice is better than white. The key is to replace processed foods with natural foods and obviously to improve our children's diets – replacing processed foods with natural, unrefined alternatives. We need to eat more fruit and vegetables, wholegrains, pulses, lean meats and low-fat dairy produce.

No Additives

Reduce or remove anything with artificial chemicals, in the form of additives, preservatives, flavours and anything else. All these put strain on the body, in particular the liver, which is so crucial for the stress response. You should try and eat lots of healthy proteins, including very lean meats, fish, poultry, cheese, yoghurt, nuts, soya products (including tofu), pulses such as lentils, seeds (three to five servings a day). Eat plenty of fruit and vegetables and their juices. Remember that the more colourful the vegetable, the more nutritious it tends to be.

Avoid the Junk

Cut down on sweets, crisps, soft drinks and fast or junk foods of any nature. These not only tend to take the place of healthier alternatives in our diet but they are also a key source of damaging chemicals, fat and anti-nutrients.

Watch the sugar! Given that stress causes the immune system to become less effective, it is important to take steps to ensure that it is being boosted in every other possible way. Sugar is one of the worst culprits in terms of immunity as it forces our bodies to work overtime in order to produce enough insulin to cope with the excess sugar, and our white blood cells are less able to fight off bacteria.

Carbohydrates and Fibre

Eat lots of carbohydrates for energy. Anything wholegrain or unrefined, including pastas, bread, brown rice, grains (such as rye, barley, corn, buckwheat), pulses, potatoes and wholegrain, sugar-free cereals. (Four to nine servings a day.)

Dietary fibre, also known as bulk or roughage, is an essential element in the diet even though it provides no nutrients. The chewing it requires stimulates saliva flow and the bulk it adds in the stomach and intestines during digestion provides more time for absorption of nutrients. It reduces the production of cholesterol and can control diabetes and weight, treat intestinal disorders and protect against cancer of the colon. The best sources of dietary fibre are fruits, vegetables, wholegrain breads, and products made from nuts and legumes. However, a diet overly abundant in dietary fibre can cut down on the absorption of important trace minerals during digestion. Take a good multi-vitamin and mineral tablet if you increase your fibre intake significantly.

Go Organic

Eat organic when you can. There is still considerable debate about whether or not it is more nutritious, but there is no doubt that it is lower in chemicals that place a strain on your system.

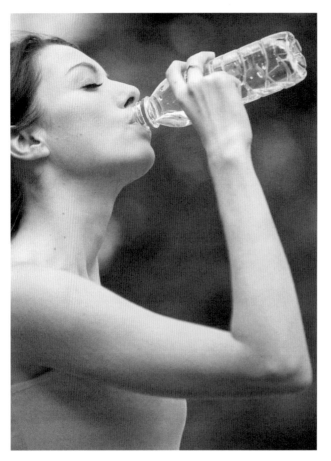

Water

About 65 per cent of our bodies are made up of water, so it is not surprising that water is the most essential element of our diets. Without food we can last for several weeks. Without water, we would be dead within a few days. Water is essential to the digestive process. If we do not drink enough between meals, the saliva flow slows down and digestion is less efficient. Almost two litres of water is excreted from our bodies every day through our skin, urine, lungs and gut, and many toxins are removed from our bodies this way. If we are losing this much water, we need to replace it.

Eliminating Toxins

The more water we drink, the greater the number of toxins eliminated. Without water our cells cannot build new tissue efficiently, toxic products build up in our blood-stream, blood volume decreases so that we have less oxygen and nutrients transported to our cells, all of which can leave us weak, tired and at risk of illness.

RDA

Three sets of figures are used to assess the adequacy of diets for the population. In the United States, a Food and Nutrition Board has been established for the purpose of determining vitamin and mineral requirements. This board is composed of distinguished scientists and nutritionists and is under the auspices of the National Academy of Sciences. Since 1940 the Board has periodically prepared a brochure listing the Recommended Dietary Allowances (RDA) of vitamins and other nutrients, based on existing knowledge. These allowances are intended as a guide for all persons involved in planning food supplies and in the interpretation of food consumption levels.

RNI

In Europe and the UK, the Reference Nutrient Intake (RNI) is used, which represents the amount of a nutrient that is deemed by the government to be sufficient to meet the needs of almost all healthy people – even those with higher than average needs. In the UK, this figure is roughly the same as the old RDA (Recommended Daily Amount), which was formerly the only set of figures used.

EAR and LRNI

The Estimated Average Requirement (EAR) is the amount of a nutrient that is considered to be sufficient to meet the needs of an average, healthy person. The Lower Reference Nutrient Intake (LRNI), represents the amount of a nutrient that is almost certain to be inadequate. For example, the average intake of the trace element selenium in the UK falls well below this figure.

Vitamins

Vitamins are compounds needed by the body in small quantities to enable us to grow, develop and function. They work with enzymes in the body, and other compounds, to help produce energy, build tissues, remove waste, and ensure that each system works effectively and efficiently. Ideally vitamins are present in roughly the same quantity in various foods.

Vitamin A

Vitamin A is a fat-soluble vitamin that comes in two forms: retinol, which is found in animal products like liver, eggs, butter and cod-liver oil, and beta-carotene, which our body converts into vitamin A when it is required. Beta-carotene is found in any brightly coloured fruit and vegetables. Beta-carotene is an antioxidant and has anticarcinogenic properties.

Sources of Vitamin A

The best sources for vitamin A are cod-liver oil, liver, kidney, eggs and dairy produce. Beta-carotene can be found in carrots, tomatoes, watercress, broccoli, spinach, cantaloupe and apricots. The RDA is believed to be inadequate, and people with special needs (e.g. following illness, suffering from infections or diabetes), should have a higher level. As vitamin A, up to 6,000 mcg can be taken if you are not pregnant. As beta-carotene, 15 mg can be taken as a preventative measure against illness. Vitamin A as retinol is toxic and should not be taken at all by pregnant women. Beta-carotene is not toxic and is considered to be safe for adults and children alike.

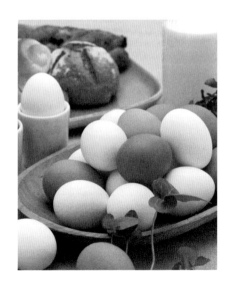

Vitamin C (Ascorbic Acid)

Vitamin C is water-soluble, which means that it is not stored by the body; we need to ensure that we get adequate amounts in our daily diets. More people take vitamin C than any other supplement and yet studies show that a large percentage of the population is still deficient.

Benefits of Vitamin C

Vitamin C is also known as ascorbic acid, and it is one of the most versatile of the vitamins needed to sustain life. It is one of the antioxidant vitamins and is believed to boost immunity and to fight cancer and infection. It reduces cholesterol and helps prevent heart disease, hastens the healing of wounds and maintains healthy bones, teeth and sex organs. Vitamin C acts as a natural antihistamine, fights cancer and helps maintain good vision.

Sources of Vitamin C

The best sources of vitamin C are rosehips, blackcurrants, broccoli, citrus fruits and is also in all fresh fruit and vegetables. At least 60 mg is necessary for health, but more is required by smokers (25 g is depleted with every cigarette), and people who are under stress, taking antibiotics, suffering from an infection, drink heavily or after an accident or injury. Daily dosages of up to 1500 mg per day appear to be safe, but take in three doses, preferably with meals and in a time-release formula. Vitamin C may cause kidney stones and gout in some people, others may suffer from diarrhoea and cramps at high dosages, although the vitamin is considered to be non-toxic at even very high levels.

Vitamin D

Vitamin D is a fat-soluble vitamin which is found in foods of animal origin, and is known as the sunshine vitamin. It can be produced in the skin from the energy of the sun, and it is not found in rich supply in any food.

Benefits of Vitamin D

Vitamin D is important for calcium and phosphorus absorption, and helps to regulate calcium metabolism. Recent research suggests that it could have a role in protecting against some cancers and infectious diseases. Deficiency is caused by inadequate exposure to sunlight, and low consumption of foods that contain vitamin D.

Sources of Vitamin D

The best sources of vitamin D are animal produce, such as milk and eggs, oily fish, butter and cheese; cod-liver oil is also a good source. Supplementation between 5–10 mcg is suggested for those at risk of deficiency. Vitamin D is the most toxic of all the vitamins, and can cause nausea, vomiting, headache and depression, among other symptoms.

Vitamin E

Vitamin E is fat-soluble and one of the key antioxidant vitamins. Its key function is as an anticoagulant, but its role in boosting the immune system and protecting against cardiovascular disease are becoming increasingly clear. Apart from its crucial antioxidant value, vitamin E is important for the production of energy and the maintenance of health at every level. Unlike most fat-soluble vitamins, vitamin E is stored in the body for only a short period of time and up to 75 per cent of the daily dose is excreted in the faeces.

Sources of Vitamin E

The best sources of vitamin E are wheatgerm (fresh), soya beans, vegetable oils, broccoli, leafy green vegetables, wholegrains, peanuts and eggs. It is available in many forms (dry is best for people with skin problems or oil intolerance). Daily dosage may be from 250–80 mg daily, but you may be advised to take higher doses in some cases. Vitamin E is non-toxic, even in high doses, but it is not suggested that you take in excess of 350 mg unless you are supervised by a registered practitioner.

Vitamin K

The K vitamins are fat-soluble and are necessary for normal blood clotting. They are often used to treat the toxic effects of anticoagulant drops, such as warfarin, and in people who have a poor ability to absorb fats.

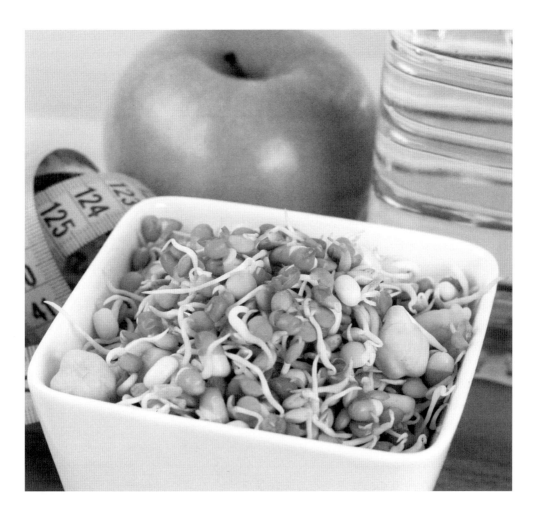

Sources of vitamin K

The best sources of Vitamin K are vegetables, such as cauliflower, spinach and peas, and wholegrain cereals. Most people produce sufficient quantities of the vitamin in the intestine, but it is estimated that we need between 500 and 1,000 mcg from our diet. There are no reports of toxicity, but because of the possibility that injected vitamin K may be related to childhood leukaemia, oral drops are suggested for newborns.

B Vitamins

There are eight B vitamins, and they play an important role in the body's metabolism, helping convert sugar to energy in the cells. They enhance the immune system and help maintain muscle tone.

B1 (Thiamine)

Thiamine is involved in all key metabolic processes in the nervous system, the heart, the blood cells and the muscle. It is useful in the treatment of nervous disorders, and can protect against imbalances caused by alcoholism. It may help to treat heart disease, anaemia, herpes and infections. It may improve mental agility and assist in controlling diabetes linked to deficiency. It helps to convert sugar to energy in the muscles and bones. Sources of B1 include all plant and animal foods, but good sources are wholegrains, brown rice, seafoods and pulses. It is also found in pork, milk, eggs, organic meats and barley.

Dosage

Heavy drinkers, smokers and women who are pregnant or taking the pill should increase normal dosage to up to 100–300 mg per day. It should be taken if you experience an increase in stressful conditions; most effective as part of a good B-complex supplement. Thiamine is non-toxic, but it is not recommended that you take more than 400 mg daily.

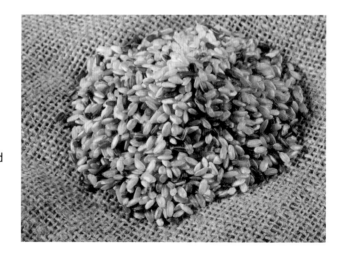

B2 (Riboflavin)

Riboflavin is a water-soluble member of the B-complex family of vitamins. It is crucial for the production of body energy and has antioxidant qualities. Riboflavin is not stored in any significant amount in the body and deficiency is common. The best sources are milk, eggs, fortified breads and cereals, green leafy vegetables and fish.

Dosage and Benefits

Riboflavin is non-toxic in most doses, but it is not recommended that you take in excess of 400 mg per day, unless supervised by a registered practitioner. It works with enzymes to metabolize fats, protein and carbohydrates. It can aid vision, promote healthy skin, hair and nails, boost athletic performance and protect against anaemia. Pregnancy, breastfeeding, taking the pill and heavy drinking all call for an increased intake.

B3 (Niacin)

Niacin takes the form of nicotinic acid and nicotinamide, and is a fairly recent addition to the family of B-complex vitamins, named as a vitamin in only 1937. Niacin has been shown to lower blood cholesterol and other body fats, and is useful in the prevention of heart disease. It may also help to prevent diabetes. It can prevent and treat schizophrenia, maintain healthy skin, tongue, nerves and digestion and reduce blood pressure.

Source of Vitamin B3

The best sources of B3 are meat, fish, wholegrain cereals, eggs, milk and cheese. Large doses may be used therapeutically, but should be taken under the supervision of a doctor or practitioner. In high doses, niacin may cause depression, liver malfunction, flushing and headaches.

B5 (Pantothenic Acid)

Pantothenic acid is a vital component of living cells. Chemical processes within the body convert it to an intermediary catalyst called coenzyme A, which is critical for the production of energy that drives cell function. It can help lower high cholesterol levels and alleviate arthritic pain.

Sources of Vitamin B5

The best sources of B5 include most grains, vegetables and meats but this vitamin is especially plentiful in liver, yeast, salmon, eggs and dairy products. It works in conjunction with all other B vitamins.

B6 (Pyridoxine)

Pyridoxine is necessary for vitamin B12 to be absorbed. B6 is required for the functioning of more than 60 enzymes in the body and is required for protein synthesis. Of all the B vitamins, B6 is the most important for a healthy immune system, and it is thought to protect the body against some types of cancer. It can help to control diabetes, assimilates proteins and fats, helps prevent skin and nervous disorders, treats the symptoms of PMS and menopause and acts as a natural diuretic.

Sources of Vitamin B6

The best sources of B6 are meat, fish, milk, eggs, wholegrain cereals and vegetables. Vitamin B6 should always be taken as part of a B-complex supplement, and in equal amounts with B1 and B2. It is toxic in high doses, causing serious nerve damage if more than 2 g per day is taken.

B9 (Folic Acid)

Folic acid is a water-soluble vitamin which forms part of the B-complex family. It is also known as vitamin Bc or vitamin B9. Low levels of folic acid may lead to anaemia. Folic acid is essential for the division of body cells, and needed for the utilization of sugar and amino acids.

Benefits of Vitamin B9

Recent findings indicate that folic acid can prevent some types of cancer and birth defects, and it is helpful in the treatment of heart disease. Most folic-acid deficiency is the result of a poor diet because it is abundant in leafy green vegetables, yeasts and liver. Taken from just before conception, and particularly in the first trimester of pregnancy, folic acid can prevent spina bifida.

Sources of Vitamin B9

The best sources are green leafy vegetables, wheatgerm, nuts, eggs, bananas, oranges and organ meats, e.g. liver. There are many people at risk of deficiency, including heavy drinkers, pregnant women, the elderly and those on low-fat diets. Supplementation at 400–800 mcg is recommended for those at risk. Take with a multivitamin and mineral supplement. Folic acid is toxic in large doses and can cause severe neurological problems.

B12 (Cobalamin)

Cobalamin is a water-soluble member of the B-complex vitamin family, and it is the only vitamin that contains essential minerals. B12 is essential for the healthy metabolism of nerve tissue and deficiencies can cause brain damage and neurological disorders. B12 may also reduce the risk of cancer and the severity of allergies, as well as boosting energy levels. Low levels of B12 result in anaemia. It promotes healthy growth in children.

Sources and Dosage

Good sources of B12 include liver, beef, pork, eggs, cheese, fish and milk. Doses of between 5–50 mcg should be adequate for most people; higher dosages should be supervised. Best taken as part of a B-complex supplement. Although Vitamin B12 is not considered to be toxic, it is not recommended that you take more than 200 mg daily, unless recommended by a registered practitioner.

Minerals

Minerals are inorganic chemical elements, which are necessary for many biochemical and physiological processes that go on in our bodies. Minerals are not necessarily present in foods: the quality of the soil and the geological conditions of the area in which they were grown play an important part in determining the mineral content of food. Even a balanced diet may be lacking in essential minerals or trace elements because of the soil in which it was grown.

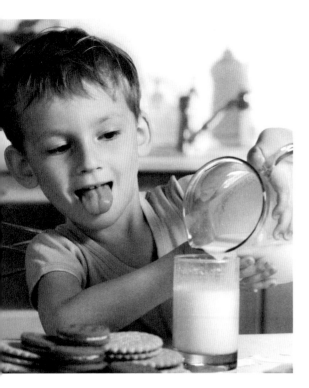

Calcium

Calcium is an important mineral, and recent research shows that we get only about one-third of what we need to maintain good health. Calcium is essential for human life – it makes up bones and teeth, and is crucial for messages to be conducted along the nerves. It ensures that our muscles contract and our hearts beat, and it is extremely important in the maintenance of the immune system, among other things.

Calcium Deficiency

There are many groups at risk of calcium deficiency – in particular the elderly – and because it is so important to body processes, our bodies take what they need from our bones, which causes them to become thin and brittle. Calcium is used therapeutically for allergies, depression, panic attacks, insomnia and hyperactivity, and extra should be taken during pregnancy and while breastfeeding. Note that doses exceeding 2,000 mg per day may cause hypercalcaemia (calcium deposits in the kidneys), but since excess calcium is excreted, it is unlikely to occur unless you are also taking excess quantities of vitamin D.

Sources of Calcium

The best sources of calcium are milk, cheese and dairy produce, leafy green vegetables, hard tap water, salmon and other tinned fish, eggs, beans, nuts and tofu. Experts recommend that calcium be taken in a good multivitamin and mineral supplement, although extra doses may be given up to 1,000 mg per day.

Potassium

Potassium is one of the most important minerals in our body, working with sodium and chloride to form electrolytes, essential body salts that make up our body fluids. Potassium is crucial for body functioning, playing a role in nerve conduction, heartbeat, energy production, synthesis of nucleic acids and proteins and muscle contraction.

Potassium Deficiency

Sweating can cause a loss of potassium, as does chronic diarrhoea and diuretics. People taking certain drugs, including corticosteroids, high-dose penicillin and laxatives, may have potassium deficiencies, and symptoms of deficiency can include vomiting, abdominal distension, muscular weakness, loss of appetite, low blood pressure and intense thirst. It activates enzymes that control energy production and improve athletic performance.

Sources of Potassium

The best sources of potassium are fresh fruit, particularly bananas, and vegetables. Eat more fresh fruit and vegetables to increase potassium intake. Diuretic users and those in a hot climate may need up to 1.5 g in supplementary potassium daily. Take them with zinc and magnesium for the best effect. In excess (doses above 17 g), potassium may cause muscular weakness and mental apathy, eventually stopping the heart.

Magnesium

Magnesium is a mineral that is absolutely essential for every biochemical process in our bodies, including metabolism and the synthesis of nucleic acids and protein. Magnesium deficiency is very common, particularly in the elderly, heavy drinkers, pregnant women and regular, strenuous exercisers, and it has been proven that even a very slight deficiency can cause a disruption of the heartbeat. Other symptoms of deficiency include weakness, fatigue, vertigo, nervousness, muscle cramps and hyperactivity in children.

Sources of Magnesium

The best sources of magnesium are brown rice, soya beans, nuts, brewer's yeast, wholewheat flour and legumes. Dietary intake is thought to be inadequate in the average Western diet; supplements of 200–400 mg are recommended daily.

Phosphorus

Phosphorus is essential to the structure and function of the body. It is present in the body as phosphates, and in this form aids the process of bone mineralization and helps to create the structure of the bone. It forms bones and teeth, produces energy and acts as a co-factor for many enzymes and activates B-complex vitamins, increasing endurance and fighting fatigue. It also forms ribonucleic acid (RNA) and deoxyribonucleic acid (DNA).

Sources of Phosphorus

The best sources of phosphorus are yeast, dried milk and milk products, wheatgerm, hard cheeses, canned fish, nuts, cereals and eggs. Phosphorus deficiency usually accompanies deficiency in potassium, magnesium and zinc, so ensure a good multivitamin and mineral supplement has all four.

Phosphorus Supplements

Supplementation should only be undertaken with supervision. Phosphorus can be toxic at dosages or intake above 1 g per day, in some cases causing diarrhoea and the calcification of organs and soft tissues, making the body unable to absorb iron, calcium, magnesium and zinc.

Iodine

Iodine is a mineral, first discovered in 1812 in kelp. Iodine was extracted and given its name because of its violet colour. It occurs naturally and is a crucial part of the thyroid hormones which monitor our energy levels.

Sources of Iodine

The best sources of iodine are seafood and seaweed, and most table salt is fortified with iodine. Optimally, iodine should be taken as potassium iodide and under the supervision of a doctor or nutritionist. Iodine is toxic in high doses and may aggravate or cause acne as large doses can interfere with hormone activity.

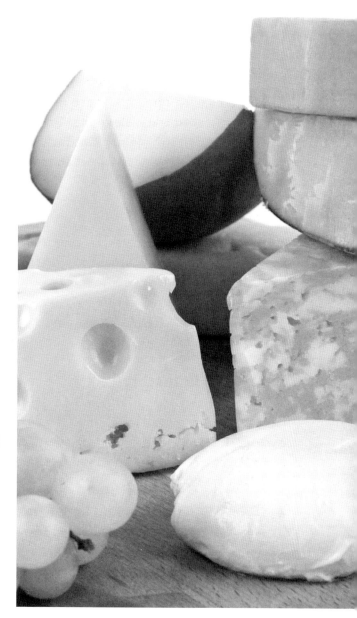

Trace Elements

Inorganic substances that are required in amounts greater than 100 mg per day are called minerals; those required in amounts less than 100 mg per day are called trace elements. Trace elements, or minerals required in quantities under 100 mg per day, include chromium, zinc, selenium, silicon, boron, copper, manganese, molybdenum, sulphur and vanadium.

Zinc

Zinc is one of the most important trace elements in our diet and it is required for more than 200 enzymic activities within the body. It is the principal protector of the immune system and is crucial in the regulation of our genetic information. Zinc is also essential for the structure and function of all cell membranes. It can prevent cancer, prevent and treat colds and stop hair loss. It is used to treat acne and other skin problems, increase male potency and treat infertility.

Effects of Zinc Deficiency

Zinc is an antioxidant and can help to detoxify the body. A zinc deficiency can cause growth failure, infertility, impotence and in some cases, an impaired sense of taste. Eczema is commonly linked to zinc deficiency: new research points to the fact that postnatal illness may be a direct result of insufficient zinc in the diet. A weakened immune system and a poor ability to heal may indicate deficiency.

Sources of Zinc

The best sources of zinc are offal, meat, mushrooms, oysters, eggs, wholegrain products and brewer's yeast. Take 15–30 mg daily, and increase copper and selenium intake if taking more zinc. Very high doses (above 150 mg per day) of zinc may cause some nausea, vomiting and diarrhoea.

Iron

Iron is required for muscle protein and is stored in the liver, spleen, bone marrow and muscles. Iron absorption is highest in childhood and reduces with age. Our bodies need vitamin C for iron to be efficiently absorbed. It improves physical performance, is anticarcinogenic, prevents learning problems in children and boosts energy levels. It can also encourage restful sleep and maintains energy levels.

Sources of Iron

The best sources of iron are shellfish, brewer's yeast, wheat bran, offal, cocoa powder, dried fruit and cereals. Pregnant, breastfeeding and menstruating women, infants, children, athletes and vegetarians may require increased levels of iron. Iron supplements will be prescribed by your doctor if necessary. Maximum dosage is 15 mg daily, unless under supervision. Excess iron can cause constipation, diarrhoea and rarely, in high doses, death.

Copper

Copper is necessary for the act of respiration – iron and copper are required for oxygen to be synthesized in the red blood cells. Copper is also important for the production of collagen, which is responsible for the health of our bones, cartilage and skin. It protects against cardiovascular disease and is useful in the treatment of arthritis. It can boost the immune system.

Dosage

Copper appears in good multivitamin and mineral supplements, and could be taken alone up to 3 mg. Excessive intake can cause vomiting, diarrhoea, muscular pain and dementia. The best sources are animal livers, shellfish, nuts, fruit, oysters, kidneys and legumes.

Selenium

Selenium is an essential trace element which has recently been recognized as one of the most important nutrients in our diet. It is an antioxidant and is vitally important to the human metabolism. Selenium has been proved to provide protection against a number of cancers and other diseases. It maintains healthy eyes and eyesight. It stimulates the immune system, improves liver function and protects against heart and circulatory diseases. Selenium can detoxify alcohol, many drugs, smoke and some fats, treat dandruff and is used in the treatment of arthritis.

Sources and Dosage

The best sources of selenium are wheatgerm, bran, tuna fish, onions, tomatoes, broccoli and wholemeal bread. Selenium supplementation should be taken with 30 to 400 IU of vitamin E to ensure that selenium works most efficiently. Selenium can be toxic in very small doses; symptoms of excess include blackened fingernails and a garlic-like odour on the breath and skin. Take no more than 500 mcg daily, unless supervised by a registered practitioner.

Fluorine

Fluorine is a trace mineral found naturally in soil, water, plants and animal tissues. Its electrically charged form is fluoride, which is how we usually refer to it. Although it has not yet been officially recognized as an essential nutrient, studies show that it is important in many processes, and may play a major role in the prevention of many modern killers, such as heart disease. It protects against dental caries, osteoporosis and may help to prevent heart disease.

Sources of Fluorine

The major source of fluorine is from drinking water, which is normally fluoridated or has enough naturally occurring fluoride to make fluoridation unnecessary. It is important that fluoride supplements are always taken with calcium. An excess of fluoride causes fluorosis, characterized by irregular patches on tooth enamel, and depresses the appetite. Eventually the spine calcifies.

Dosage

The typical daily intake is 1–2 mg. Tablets and drops are available from pharmacies, but should be limited to 1 mg daily in adults and 0.25–0.5 mg for children. Do not supplement fluoride without the advice of your dentist.

Cobalt

Cobalt is a constituent of vitamin B12. The amount of cobalt you have in your body is dependent on the amount of cobalt in the soil and therefore in the food we eat. Most of us are not deficient in cobalt, although deficiency is much more common in vegetarians. With vitamin B12 cobalt can prevent pernicious anaemia, help in the production of red blood cells, aid in the synthesis of DNA and choline, encourage a healthy nervous system, reduce blood pressure and help with the maintenance of myelin, the fatty sheath that protects the nerves.

Sources of Cobalt

The best sources of cobalt are fresh leafy, green vegetables, meat, liver, milk, oysters and clams. Cobalt is rarely found in supplement form, but makes up part of a good multivitamin and mineral supplement with the B-complex vitamins; 8 mcg daily appears to be adequate.

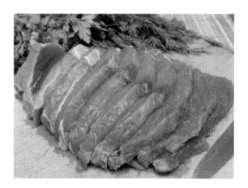

Boron

Recent research has reported that boron added to the diets of post-menopausal women prevented calcium loss and bone demineralization – a revolutionary discovery for sufferers of osteoporosis. It is also claimed that boron will raise testosterone levels and build muscle in men and is therefore often used by athletes and body builders. Boron is found in most fruit and vegetables, and does not appear in meat and meat products. Boron supplements are usually taken in the form of sodium borate.

Dosage

Boron can be toxic, with symptoms including a red rash, vomiting, diarrhoea, reduced circulation, shock and coma. A fatal dose is 15–20 g, 3–6 g in children. Symptoms appear at about 100 mg. There is no Recommended Daily Allowance (RDA), but it is suggested that you take 3 mg daily to prevent osteoporosis.

Molybdenum

Molybdenum is a vital part of the enzyme responsible for the utilization of iron in our bodies. Molybdenum may also be an antioxidant and recent research indicates that it is necessary for optimum health.

Benefits of Molybdenum

Molybdenum can help prevent anaemia and is known to promote a feeling of well-being. A deficiency may result in dental caries, sexual impotence in men and cancer of the gullet. Deficiency is usually the result of eating foods from molybdenum-deficient soils, or a diet that is high in refined and processed foods.

Dosage

Molybdenum is toxic in doses higher than 10–15 mg, which causes gout (a build-up of uric acid around the joints). The best sources are wheat, canned beans, wheatgerm, liver, pulses, wholegrains, offal and eggs. The optimal intake is still undecided; adequate amounts are between 0.075–0.25 mg per day, but intake will differ between individuals. Experts suggest 50–100 mcg per day as a preventative measure.

Chromium

Chromium is an important regulator of blood sugar and has been used successfully in the control and treatment of diabetes. It is involved in the metabolism of carbohydrates and fats and is used in the production of insulin in the body.

High levels of sugars in the diet cause chromium to be excreted through the kidneys; it is important that you get enough in your diet if you eat sugary foods. The incidence of diabetes and heart disease decreases with increased levels of chromium in the body.

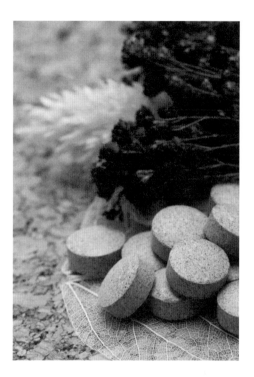

Sources and Dosage

The best sources of chromium are wholegrain cereals, meat and cheese, brewer's yeast, molasses and egg yolk. There is no Recommended Daily Allowance (RDA), but it is suggested that 25 mcg per day is adequate. Supplements up to 200 mcg per day may be appropriate.

Manganese

Manganese is necessary for the normal functioning of the brain, and effective in the treatment of many nervous disorders, including Alzheimer's disease and schizophrenia. Deficiency is usually related to a poor diet – particularly one where foods are processed and refined.

Manganese Deficiency

There is some evidence that diabetes, heart disease and schizophrenia are linked to manganese deficiency. Toxic levels are usually quite rare, but symptoms of excess manganese may include lethargy, involuntary movements, posture problems and coma.

Sources and Dosage

The best sources are cereals, tea, green leaf vegetables, wholemeal bread, pulses and nuts. A dosage of 2–5 mg is considered adequate, but doses up to 10 mg are thought to be safe.

Antioxidants

Much of the cell damage that occurs in disease is caused by highly destructive chemical groups known as free radicals. These are the products of oxidation, a process that naturally occurs in our body as we breathe. Today, because of increasing levels of pollution in the air, there are more free radicals than ever before. In small quantities free radicals can fight off bacteria and viruses, but in larger quantities they encourage the ageing process and cause premature damage to our cells.

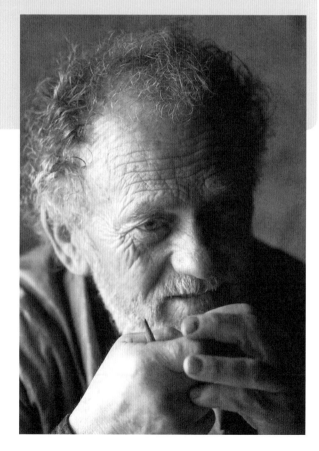

Free Radicals

Free-radical damage is believed to be the basis for the ageing process and for the visible signs of ageing, such as greying hair, wrinkles, skin changes and muscle wastage. Free radicals can be formed by exposure to radiation and toxic chemicals, such as those found in cigarette smoke, over-exposure to the sun's rays or various metabolic processes, such as the process of breaking down stored fat molecules for use as an energy source.

Controlling Free Radicals

Free radicals are normally kept in check by the action of free-radical scavengers which occur naturally in the body and which act to neutralize the free radicals. The body makes these as a matter of course. There are also a number of nutrients that act as antioxidants, including vitamin A, beta-carotene, vitamins C and E and the minerals selenium and zinc.

Sources of Antioxidants

Although many antioxidants can be obtained from food sources, such as fresh fruit and vegetables, it is difficult to get enough of them from these sources to prevent the generation of free radicals caused by our polluted environment, the number of chemicals in our foods and many other factors. Free-radical damage can be minimized by taking supplements of key nutrients such as alpha-lipoic acid, bilberry, coenzyme Q10, cysteine, grapeseed extract, Ginkgo biloba, glutathione and green tea.

Many trials have shown that additional antioxidant vitamins, such as 2,000 mg of C and 400 mg of E daily, can significantly reduce the number of heart attacks, strokes, cataracts and other diseases, and slow down the process of ageing. The following also represents promising research.

Vitamin E

Vitamin E has been found to enhance a variety of immune-system responses by reducing blood stickiness, the harmful effects of toxins such as cigarette smoke, the damage caused by the sun (when applied topically) and halving the risk of heart attack in those with heart disease. Vitamin E also prevents cataracts and, when taken with vitamin A, improves some cases of hearing loss. It is essential for skin health, and age spots are one of the key deficiency signs.

Selenium

Selenium is the other most important antioxidant and it has now been proven that it decreases the rate of cancer and increases life span. Selenium deficiency is also signalled by age spots, cataracts, cancerous changes, infections, muscle inflammation and heart disease, so it has an undoubted effect on many parts of the body. In research studies, selenium supplements have been found to improve kidney function, help prevent liver cancer, enhance immune function, improve thyroid function, treat skin conditions and reduce the symptoms of arthritis.

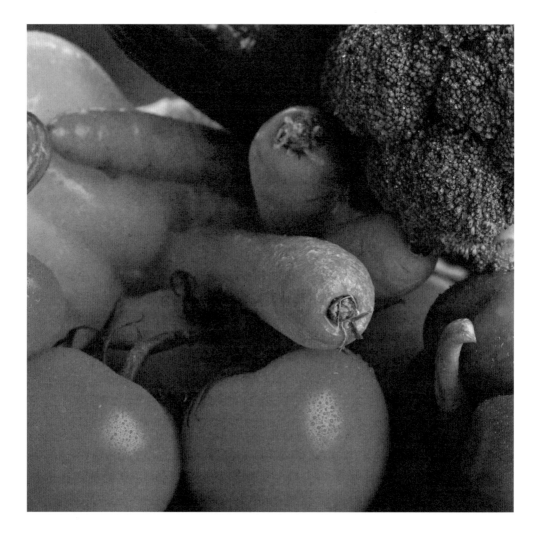

Beta-carotene

Beta-carotene is known as a carotenoid and is a precursor to vitamin A. It has antioxidant properties, and when food or supplements containing beta-carotene are consumed, the beta-carotene is converted to vitamin A by the liver. According to recent reports, beta-carotene appears to help prevent cancer by neutralizing free radicals. Taking large amounts of vitamin A over a long period of time can be toxic, but no such overdose can occur with beta-carotene. It prevents and treats skin disorders and ageing of the skin, improves vision and prevents night blindness and improves the body's ability to heal.

The best sources of beta-carotene are any brightly coloured fruits and vegetables, such as carrots, tomatoes, watercress, broccoli, spinach, cantaloupe and apricots. The Recommended Daily Allowance (RDA) is now believed to be inadequate, and people with special needs (following illness, suffering from infections, with diabetes, for example), should have a higher level: 15,000 iu is considered to be the optimum dose.

Bioflavonoids

Bioflavonoids were originally called vitamin P, and are also known as flavones. They accompany vitamin C in natural foods and are responsible for the colour in the leaves, flowers and stems of food plants. Their primary job is to protect the capillaries, keep them strong and prevent bleeding. The best sources are citrus fruits, apricots, cherries, green peppers, broccoli and lemons. The central white core of citrus fruits is the richest source.

Properties

Many of the medicinally active substances of herbs are bioflavonoids, which are non-toxic, and should be taken with vitamin C for best effect. Bioflavonoids reduce bruising in susceptible individuals, protect capillaries, protect against cerebral and other haemorrhaging, and reduce menstrual bleeding. They have antioxidant properties, and encourage vitamin C's own antioxidant qualities.

Amino Acids

Amino acids are organic compounds that comprise the building-blocks of proteins in the body. A number of amino acids play an essential role in building our bodies. There are many different amino acids, about 20 of which are the main constituents of proteins; only about half of these are classified as essential nutrients, that is, necessary in the human diet.

Role of Amino Acids in the Body

Proteins are essential substances in our diets because of their constituent amino acids. Nutritionally, complete proteins are those that contain the right concentrations of amino acids which humans cannot synthesize from other amino acids or other sources. An adequate diet, however, may be achieved by consuming the correct mixture of proteins, some of which might be deficient in one amino acid but rich in another. Some of these amino acids are used directly as building-blocks in the synthesis of new proteins, while others may be used to supply energy and still others, particularly when large amounts of proteins are consumed, may be excreted in urine. Amino acids are necessary to make almost all elements in the body, including hair, skin, bone, tissue, antibodies, hormones, enzymes and blood.

Phenylalanine

L-Phenylalanine is an essential amino acid, necessary for a number of biochemical processes, including the synthesis of neurotransmitters in the brain. It is said to promote sexual arousal and to release hormones that help to control appetite. It can help to alleviate depression and control addictive behaviour. It also reduces hunger and cravings for food.

Sources and Dosage

The best sources of phenylalanine are proteins, cheese, almonds, peanuts, sesame seeds and soya. L-Phenylalanine is usually available in 500 mg doses. Take on an empty stomach for best effect and do not take with protein. If you suffer from skin cancer, do not take L-Phenylalanine. People with high blood pressure should only take supplementary L-Phenylalanine with their

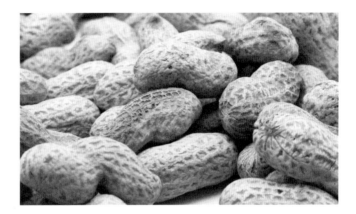

doctor's supervision. It is not suitable for use with monoamine oxidase inhibitors (MAOI) antidepressants. Pregnant women should not take this amino acid.

Tryptophan

This essential amino acid is used by the brain, along with several vitamins and minerals, to produce serotonin, a neurotransmitter. Serotonin, which regulates and induces sleep, is also said to reduce sensitivity to pain. It was one of the first amino acids to be produced for sale as a supplement, and it is useful as a natural sleeping aid. It may help to encourage sleep and prevent jet lag. It can also reduce sensitivity to pain and cravings for alcohol. It is a natural antidepressant and may help to reduce anxiety and panic attacks.

Sources and Dosage

The best sources of tryptophan are cottage cheese, milk, meat, fish, turkey, bananas and proteins. Used to prevent panic attacks and depression, it should be taken between meals with juice or water (no proteins). To help induce sleep, take 500 mg along with vitamin B6, niacinamide and magnesium an hour or so before bedtime. There is some evidence that tryptophan may cause liver problems in high doses, and although studies vary, it is now believed that it can be toxic in very high doses. Take only with the advice of your doctor.

Lysine

Lysine is an essential amino acid, which means that it is necessary for life. It is needed for growth, tissue repair, and for the production of antibodies, hormones and enzymes. It should be obtained from the diet, although supplements are available. Lysine is not suitable for children. High doses are now believed to be effective in reducing the recurrence of outbreaks of herpes. It may help to build muscle mass, prevent fertility problems and improve concentration.

Sources and Dosage

The best sources of lysine are fish, milk, lima beans, meat, cheese, yeast, eggs and all proteins. Up to 500 g daily is believed to be safe, although some experts recommend 1 g daily at mealtimes. Take on an empty stomach, with some juice or water; do not mix with other proteins. Take with an equal quantity of arginine if you want to increase muscle mass.

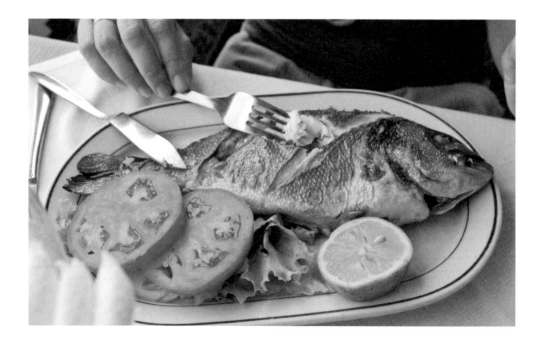

Cysteine

The amino acid cysteine contains sulphur, which is said to work as an antioxidant, protecting and preserving the cells in our body. It is also said to protect the body against pollutants, but much work has still to be done to properly understand the effects of cysteine. It may protect against copper toxicity and protects the body against free radicals and may help reverse the damage done by smoking and alcohol abuse. It offers protection against X-rays and nuclear radiation.

Sources and Dosage

The best source of cysteine are eggs, meat, dairy products and some cereals. Take with vitamin C for best effect (three times as much vitamin C as cysteine); doses up to 1 g are considered to be safe. Diabetics should not take cysteine supplements unless supervised by their doctor. Cysteine may also cause kidney stones but a high vitamin C intake should prevent this from occurring.

Methionine

Methionine is a sulphur-containing amino acid that is very important in numerous processes in the body. Research shows that it may help to prevent clogging of the arteries by eliminating fatty substances. The best sources of methionine are eggs, milk, liver and fish.

Benefits of Methionine

Methionine may help to eliminate fatty substances in the blood and help to regulate the nervous system. In conjunction with choline and folic acid, it may prevent some tumours. It is necessary for the biosynthesis of taurine and cysteine. Supplements are not advised, although some doctors may suggest their use in specific circumstances.

Arginine

L-arginine is one of the most important and useful amino acids, with a significant role in muscle growth and repair, helping to regulate and support key components of the immune system. It is also extremely important for male fertility.

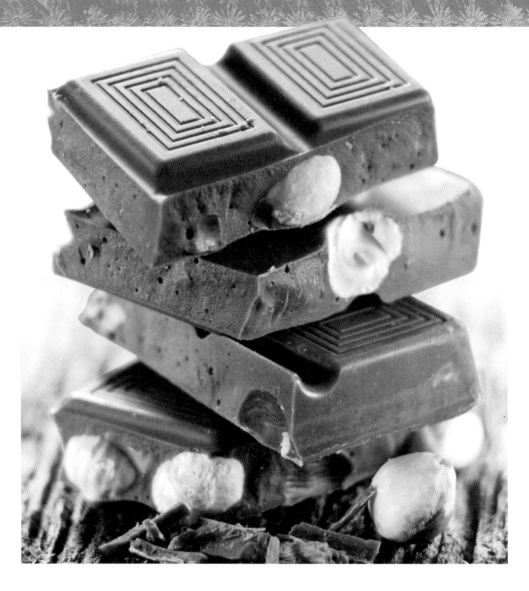

A non-essential amino acid, it is capable of being synthesized in the body and it is therefore not crucial that we get additional amounts in our daily diet. It is, however, essential for children. It can fight cancer by inhibiting the growth of tumours and helps protect the liver and detoxify harmful substances. It can also increase a low sperm count in men.

Sources and Dosage

The best sources are raw cereals, chocolate and nuts. The optimal intake is unknown, but doses of up to 1.5 g appear to be safe. Take arginine with lysine, which inhibits herpes attacks in carriers. Take on an empty stomach and avoid consuming in excess as it could cause mental and metabolic disturbances, nausea and diarrhoea. Prolonged high doses may be dangerous to children and to anyone with liver or kidney problems.

Carnitine

L-carnitine is a non-essential amino acid, which is necessary for many functions in the body, the most important of which is its role in regulating fat metabolism – in other words, transporting fat across membranes to the energy burning parts of cells. The more carnitine available, the faster the fat is transported, and the more fat is used for energy. Recent studies show that carnitine may be useful in the treatment of some forms of heart disease and in muscular dystrophy. Food sources of carnitine include meats and dairy foods.

Dosage

L-carnitine supplementation is believed to be safe between 1.5–2 g daily, although experts recommend that you only take it for one week a month; 500 mg daily is thought to be adequate dosage for improving athletic performance.

Taurine

Taurine is a non-essential amino acid that is produced by the body. Its main role is to regulate the nerves and muscle and help to co-ordinate neurotransmission. Studies performed on animals show that a diet low in taurine can cause degeneration of the retina and impaired vision.

Sources and Dosage

Good sources of taurine are meat, fish and eggs, but none of the plant foods. An excessive intake of taurine can cause depression and other symptoms. Doses of up to 3 g are used to treat high blood pressure, epilepsy and other conditions relating to the eyes; 50–100 mg is usually prescribed, taken two to three times a week.

Aspartic Acid

L-Aspartic acid is a non-essential amino acid that has been used for many years in the treatment of chronic fatigue. Studies confirm the efficiency of this amino acid in raising energy levels and in helping to overcome the side effects of drug withdrawal. Do not take with protein, such as milk, and do not take more than 1 g without the supervision of your doctor. Supplements are available in 250–500 mg tablets; take three times daily with juice or water.

Glycine

Glycine is considered to be the simplest of the amino acids, with a variety of properties that are still being studied. It is good for low pituitary-gland function. Glycine can be used in the treatment of spastic movement – particularly in patients suffering from multiple sclerosis and to treat progressive muscular dystrophy. It is also used in the treatment of hypoglycaemia. It is not recommended that you take this amino acid as a supplement unless supervised by your doctor. Doses below 1 g are thought to be safe, but research is ongoing.

Dimethylglycine (DMG)

Dimethylglycine is a derivative of glycine, the simplest of the amino acids. It acts as a building block for many important substances, including a number of important hormones, neurotransmitters and DNA. Choose supplements produced by a reputable supplier, and follow the instructions on the label. Do not exceed the recommended dose.

Benefits of DMG

Low levels of DMG are present in meats, seeds and grains. No deficiency symptoms are associated with a lack of DMG in the diet, but taking supplemental DMG can have a wide range of therapeutic benefits, including helping the body to maintain high energy levels and boosting mental acuity. DMG has also been found to enhance the immune system, and to reduce elevated blood cholesterol. It helps to normalize blood pressure and blood-sugar levels and improves the functioning of many organs.

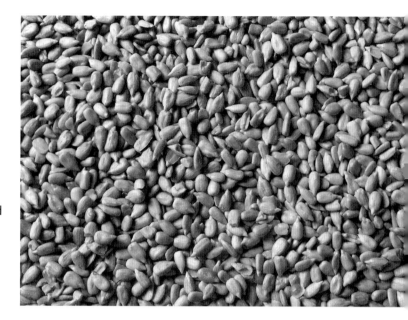

Histadine

Histadine is one of the lesser-known amino acids, and its role in our bodies is not yet fully understood. Research is ongoing into the possible effects of histadine supplementation. It is used in the treatment of arthritis and for those who have an abnormally low level of this amino acid in their blood. It may boost the activity of suppressor T-cells, which could be useful in the fight against AIDS and auto-immune conditions. Do not take more than 1.5 g daily unless supervised by your doctor.

Glutamine

Glutamine is a derivative of glutamic acid, which is believed to help reduce cravings for alcohol. Studies are inconclusive as to the real benefits of taking this amino acid, and it is not recommended that you take more than 1 g daily unless you are supervised by a doctor. It can help reduce craving for alcohol, speed the healing of peptic ulcers, relieve depression, energize the mind and may help to treat and prevent colitis.

Essential Fatty Acids

Essential fatty acids are not only crucial to health, but are a form of healthy fat, which our obsession with a fat-free diet has nearly eliminated. Essential fatty acids are converted into substances that keep our blood thin, lower blood pressure, decrease inflammation, improve the function of our nervous and immune systems, help insulin to work, affect our vision, co-ordination and mood, encourage healthy metabolism and maintain the balance of water in our bodies.

Types of Fatty Acids

Fatty acids fall into two main categories: omega-3 and omega-6 oils. Omega-3 oils are found in leafy green vegetables, pumpkin seeds, flaxseed oil, walnuts and oily fish (including salmon, herring, sardines, mackerel, pilchards and fresh tuna). Omega-6 oils are found in vegetables and seed oils (including corn, soya, sesame, sunflower and safflower oils) and in peanuts, peanut oils and olive oils.

Using Oils

Choose cold-pressed olive oil for cooking, which does not become unstable when heated. Add flaxseed oil (available as capsules or as an oil on its own), which has the highest concentration of omega-3 oils, to your diet; it should not be heated, but you can drizzle a little in salads, or add it to yoghurts or warm foods just before serving.

Fish Oils

A source of essential fatty acids (EFAs), fish oils contain two long-chain fatty acids called eicosopentaenoic acid (EPA) and docosahexaenoic acid (DHA), which affect the synthesis of prostaglandins, which in turn have a regulatory effect on the body. There are numerous claims for fish oils, which are now believed to improve overall health and treat many conditions. They may be useful in the treatment of kidney disease, and can counteract the effects of some immunosuppressive drugs. They may help to prevent cancer, in particular breast cancer. Fish oils can stop the progression of arthritis and can protect against high blood pressure.

Sources and Usage

The best sources of fish oils are herring, salmon, tuna, cod and prawns. Fish oils may be harmful to diabetics by causing an increase in blood-sugar levels and a decline in insulin secretion. People suffering from arthritis or psoriasis can take up to 4 g daily, but for most people it is most suitable to increase your intake of fish and seafood in order to achieve the benefits of the fish oils in the natural form. Maximum suggested dosage for supplements, without the supervision of your doctor, is 900 mg per day.

Flaxseed Oil *(Linum usitatissimum)*

The seeds of the flax plant contain a remarkable healing oil which can be used both internally and externally. Flaxseed is also known as linseed, but should not be confused with the boiled linseed oil available from building merchants.

Applications

As far back as Hippocrates, flaxseed tea has been used to treat sore throats, hoarseness and the spasms of bronchitis. Flaxseed is a rich source of essential fatty acids (EFAs), and supplementing with flaxseed is one of the best ways to ensure an oil balance in your diet. Flaxseed is mildly laxative and is a good tonic for the kidneys and encourages their action. It is analgesic and antispasmodic. Apply the oil to sprains to reduce inflammation and ease the pain. Mix with lime water to reduce the pain of burns.

Tea

Flaxseed (linseed) tea can be used for mild constipation, and to encourage kidney function; the tea also works to ease kidney pains and cramping. The tea can be drunk during bouts of bronchitis to reduce the inflammation of the lungs and prevent spasm. Take the supplement for all the health benefits associated with EFAs.

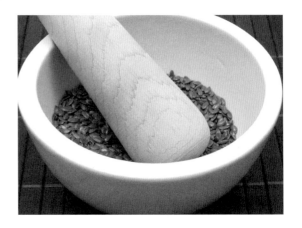

Evening Primrose Oil *(Oenothera biennis)*

Native Americans were the first to recognize the potential of evening primrose oil as a healer, and they decocted (boiled) the seeds to make a liquid for healing wounds. Evening primrose oil is a rich source of gamma linolenic acid, which is better known as GLA.

The body makes GLA from essential fatty acids (EFAs). EFAs have numerous functions in the body – one of which is to manufacture hormone-like substances called prostaglandins, which have very important effects on the body, such as toning blood vessels, balancing water levels, aiding the action of the digestive system and brain functioning. Prostaglandins also have a beneficial effect on the immune system.

Uses

It reduces scaling and redness, prevents itching and encourages healing in cases of eczema; it is also used in the treatment of psoriasis. It discourages dry skin and ensures that the cellular membranes that make up the skin are stable and strong; there is some evidence that the oil retards the ageing process. Evening primrose oil may help to prevent multiple sclerosis (MS) and appears to be particularly useful for children suffering from the condition.

It may help in cases of liver damage caused by alcohol (cirrhosis of the liver), hyperactivity in children and cystic fibrosis. It has a stimulating effect on the body, encouraging it to convert fat into energy, making it an excellent treatment for obesity. Hormonal imbalances, perhaps causing conditions like PMS, and symptoms of the menopause may be eased by reducing symptoms of bloating, water retention, irritability and depression.

Dosage

Evening primrose oil is most often taken in the form of capsules, but it is also available as an oil (sometimes flavoured), and it can be applied to the skin to treat skin conditions. Take 500 mg each day for two months and then for the 10 days preceding each period if you suffer from PMS.

In menopause, 2,000–4,000 mg should be taken daily for four weeks and then 500–1,000 mg daily thereafter. For asthma, take two 500 mg tablets, three times daily for three to four months, and then one tablet three times daily. If you are taking steroids, this treatment will not work because steroids interfere with the action of evening primrose oil.

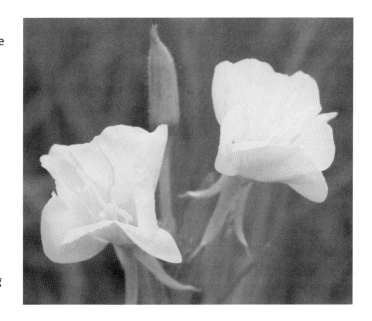

Supplements

Supplements are elements of nutrition that are given supplementally. There is a wide range of vitamins, minerals and other substances available in supplement form, but there are also a number of food supplements that do not fall strictly within the definitions of vitamins, minerals, lipids and amino acids. These include various elements that either have healing properties or are now known to be crucial to health.

Understanding Supplements

Supplements are not a replacement for food, and they cannot be ingested without food. Supplements are no substitute for a poor diet, but they will enhance a good one. People suffering from chronic conditions or who smoke or drink regularly may need to take supplements to ensure optimum health.

It is important to remember that micronutrients work in conjunction with one another, and taking large doses of any one supplement can upset the balance within the body. A good vitamin and mineral supplement will ensure that you are getting the correct amounts of each, according to the relationships between them. Extra supplements should only be taken on the advice of a registered nutritionist or medical practitioner. Where supplements are taken to discourage the course of illness – for example, vitamin C for colds or flu – it is safe to take larger doses than usual. Read the packet for further information.

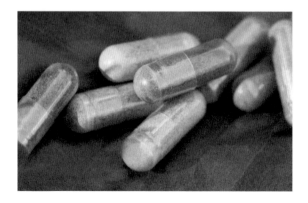

Taking Supplements

The best time for taking most supplements is after meals, on a full stomach, although some vitamins and minerals work best on an empty stomach. Read the label on any supplement you plan to take to find out the best time to take it.

Time-release formulas need to be taken with food, for their nutrients are slowly released over a period of hours. If there is not enough food to slow their passage through the body, they can pass the sites where they are normally absorbed before they have had a chance to release their nutrients. Take supplements evenly throughout the day for best effect.

Lecithin

Lecithin has for some time been a popular supplement, used for a variety of health conditions. It comprises choline, insoitol, fatty acids and phosphorus and is available as a liquid or as dry granules. It is widely used in foods to maintain consistency, and is one of the only nutritious food additives. Lecithin protects against cardiovascular disease and helps to reduce high blood pressure. It is used to treat memory loss and nervous conditions such as dementia and Alzheimer's disease. It may also help in the treatment of mental disorders such as manic depression.

Sources and Dosage

The best sources are egg yolks, soya beans, liver, meats, fish, cauliflower and cabbage. Doses of up to 1 g daily are acceptable, but see your doctor to discuss your individual needs. Lecithin appears in a wide range of foods and it is probably best to increase your intake of these instead of supplementing. Lecithin in large quantities may cause depression in some people. Very high doses may even cause nausea, vomiting and dizziness.

Ginkgo Biloba

Ginkgo biloba is one of the most widely sold herbs in Europe, typically taken for cognitive enhancement, circulatory disorders, and as a powerful antioxidant. An ever-increasing range of

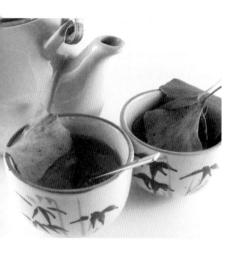

research is being undertaken into its therapeutic qualities, and the results have been nothing short of amazing.

Benefits

Ginkgo has been one of the most commonly prescribed herbs in the Chinese *materia medica* for over 5,000 years, and it has been used to treat a huge range of conditions, including age-related circulation and memory loss, cancer, asthma, pulmonary diseases, impaired hearing and sexual dysfunction. It improves blood flow, strengthens blood vessels, is anti-inflammatory and relaxes the lungs.

It aids poor circulation, thrombosis, varicose veins, cramp which comes on walking, white finger and spontaneous bruising. It is especially helpful for failing circulation to the brain in elderly people and often improves deafness, tinnitus, vertigo and early senile dementia.

Bee and Flower Pollen

In flowering plants the pollen-producing spores are located in the stamens of flowers. Flower pollen is said to be purer than bee pollen. Bee pollen is found in the hives themselves. It is rich in protein and amino acids and, along with honey, forms the basic diet of all the bees in the hive, except for the queen. Pollen has been used as medicine around the world for thousands of years.

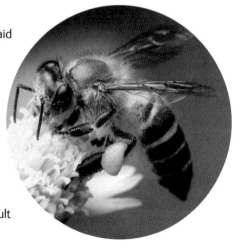

If you suffer from hay fever or are allergic to bee stings you may suffer a reaction to bee pollen. Consult with your doctor before taking this supplement.

Sources and Dosage

The best source is unpasteurized honey, which contains small amounts of bee pollen. It can help to suppress appetite and cravings, may improve skin problems and retard the ageing process, and could help with prostate problems. It is also good for regulating the bowels. Daily 400 mg doses appear to be safe levels. Always take pollen with food.

Kelp

Kelp is a type of seaweed, which is a rich source of vitamins, particularly B vitamins, and many valuable minerals and trace elements. True kelps belong to the genus *laminaria*, such as *Laminaria digitata* (oarweed), but there are several genera and varieties. Kelp can be beneficial to the brain tissue, the membranes surrounding the brain, the sensory nerves and the spinal cord. It helps with the health of the nails and blood vessels and is used in the treatment of thyroid problems because of its high iodine content. Kelp is useful for other conditions, such as hair loss, obesity and ulcers. It protects against the effects of radiation and softens stools.

Kelp is available in a wide variety of forms including raw, dried, granulated, powdered or even liquid. It can be taken as a daily dietary supplement, particularly in people with mineral deficiencies.

Acidophilus

Acidophilus (also known as *Lactobacillus acidophilus*) is a source of friendly intestinal bacteria (flora). Healthy bacteria play an important role in our bodies, and unless they are continually supplied with some form of lactic acid or lactose (such as Acidophilus) can die, causing a host of health problems. Many doctors and health practitioners recommend taking Acidophilus alongside oral antibiotics, which can cause diarrhoea, destroy the healthy flora of the intestines and lead to fungal infections. Acidophilus may also help to ensure vaginal health. The best sources are natural, unflavoured and live yoghurt.

Further Reading

Bach, Edward, *Heal Thyself* (C.W. Daniel Company, 1978)

Bach, Edward, *The Twelve Healers and Other Remedies* (C.W. Daniel Company, 1973)

Brinker, Francis *et al*, *Herb Contraindications and Drug Interactions* (2nd edition) (Electric Medical Publications, 1998)

Cosway-Hayes, Joan, *Reflexology For Everybody* (Footloose Press, 1999)

Forem, Jack & Shimer, Steve, *Healing with Pressure Point Therapy: Simple, Effective Techniques for Massaging Away More Than 100 Common Ailments* (Prentice Hall Press, 1999)

Frangles, Nora, *Simple Guide to Using Acupuncture* (Global Books Ltd., 2000)

Johari, Harish, *Ayurvedic Massage: Traditional Indian Techniques for Balancing Body and Mind* (Inner Traditions International Ltd., 1996)

Johnson, Maria, Donna & Coles, *Making Aromatherapy Creams and Lotions: 101 Natural Remedies to Revitalize and Nourish Your Skin* (Storey Books, 2000)

Lavery, Sheila & Ness, Caro, *Aromatherapy: A Step-by-Step Guide* (Element, 1997)

Lee, Helen, *Tao of Beauty: Chinese Herbal Secrets to Feeling Good and Looking Great* (Bantam Books Paperback, 1999)

Lubeck, Walter, *The Complete Reiki Handbook* (Lotus Light, 1995)

Master Hong Lui, *The Healing Art of Qi Gong* (Time Warner International, 1999)

Miller, Lucinda M. (Ed.) & Murray, Wallace J. (Ed.), *Herbal Medicinals: A Clinician's Guide* (Haworth, 1995)

Murray, Michael, T. & Pizzorno, Joseph E., *The Encyclopedia of Natural Medicine* (2nd Ed.) (Prima Publishing Paperback, 1997)

Ody, P., *The Herb Society's Complete Medicinal Herbal* (Dorling Kindersley, 1992)

Seem, Mark, *A New American Acupuncture: Acupuncture Osteopathy: The Myofascial Release of the Body's Mind* (Blue Poppy Press, 1993)

Vennells, David, *Reiki for Beginners* (Llewellyn Publications, 2000)

Websites

www.abchomeopathy.com
Great website for learning the basics of homeopathic medicine, including a forum.

www.acufinder.com
Find an acupuncturist in almost any country.

www.aromatherapy.com
US-based company that ships essential oils internationally.

www.aromatherapycouncil.co.uk
Gives advice on how to become a professional aromatherapist and more information on aromatherapy.

www.aromaweb.com
Has an index of aromatherapy recipes and a link to an aromatherapy blog.

www.boiron.com
Boiron makes both preventative cures and homeopathic remedies that can be taken during the illness.

www.eatwell.gov.uk/healthydiet
Provides a diagram of what a person should eat and how much of it. Also has a comprehensive breakdown of all the vitamins and minerals that make up a balanced diet.

www.grannymed.com
Has home remedies for dozens of various ailments as well as an 'Ask the Expert' forum where questions can be directed to a practising nurse.

www.herbnet.com
This website has forums to ask herbalists for advice as well as a 'Herbalpedia' available for purchase with information on over 2,300 different botanicals.

www.homeopathic.com
Offers a place to purchase books dedicated to homeopathy as well as advice on what remedy will work best for an ailment.

www.homeopathic.org
This website provides ways to connect with professional homeopaths in addition to a list of trusted homeopathic remedy suppliers in both the US and Canada.

www.medicinalhoney.com.au
This site offers a place to buy honey with markedly high levels of phytoactivity, as well as honey skin care products.

www.natural-homeremedies.com
Natural home remedies for various ailments.

www.naturopathyonline.com
Provides naturopathic remedies for various ailments and recipes for healthy meals to prevent future illness.

www.nutritiondata.com
Offers various diets targeted at health issues such as diabetes and heart problems. Can also analyse recipes.

www.thedance.com/herbs/ayurveda.htm
A breakdown of the Ayurvedic school of herbalism that includes a chart to determine which dosha or doshas are strongest in a person.

www.xynergy.co.uk
Has pages dedicated to different types of herbal remedies.

www.yogajournal.com
Website for beginning and advanced yoga enthusiasts alike. Site includes poses, words of wisdom and a directory of yoga instructors.

www.youraromatherapy.co.uk
UK-based company that ships essential oils as well as diffusers internationally.

Index